Mosby's

NURSING
PDQ

FOR
MEDICATION SAFETY

Practical · Detailed · Quick

Prepared by the
Institute for
Safe Medication Practices

Consultants
Evelyn Salerno,
RPh, BS, PharmD

D1374307

MOSBY

ELSEVIER
MOSBY

11830 Westline Industrial Drive
St. Louis, Missouri 63146

Mosby's Nursing PDQ for Medication Safety   ISBN 0-323-03139-

Copyright © 2005, Mosby, Inc. All rights reserved.

NOTICE

Health care is an ever-changing field. Standard safety precautions must
be followed, but as new research and clinical experience broaden our
knowledge, changes in treatment and drug therapy may become
necessary or appropriate. Readers are advised to check the most
current product information provided by the manufacturer of each drug
to be administered to verify the recommended dose, the method and
duration of administration, and contraindications. It is the
responsibility of the licensed prescriber, relying on experience and
knowledge of the patient, to determine dosages and the best treatment
for each individual patient. Neither the publisher nor the editor
assumes any liability for any injury and/or damage to persons or
property arising from this publication.

The Publisher

Senior Acquisitions Editor: Tom Wilhelm
Senior Developmental Editor: Lauren Borstell
Publishing Services Manager: Gayle May
Project Manager: JoAnn Amore
Cover Design: Julia Dummitt

MW/C&C

Printed in China

Last digit is the print number : 9 8 7 6 5 4 3 2

Primum non nocere. Above all, do no harm. Nurses and other healers have lived by this motto for hundreds of years. The minimum our patients expect from us and deserve to receive is safe and compassionate care. But in today's complex world of medicine, our best intentions can have unintended and sometimes harmful consequences.

Sadly, medication errors are one of the most common ways in which patients are harmed despite our best intentions. As nurses, we administer medications to patients with the intention to improve health and well-being, promote healing, and reduce suffering. Unfortunately, this tremendous responsibility is fraught with inherent risks. Despite our most caring, competent, and vigilant practice, medication errors happen every day, to every type of healthcare provider, in every type of healthcare setting. The bad news: errors will continue to happen because we are human. The good news: there are ways that you can reduce the risk of making errors and minimize the potential for harm to your patients.

Mosby's Nursing PDQ for Medication Safety is a quick resource manual to help you protect your patients from harm. It was created to give you practical information, at your fingertips, to reduce the risk of making a serious medication error. While it is NOT a typical drug reference all about specific medications, *Mosby's Nursing PDQ for Medication Safety* offers many informative lists, charts, and tables, topics for discussion, and self-assessment questions, all intended to:

- Increase your knowledge of the causes of medication errors
- Encourage you to think about medication errors as a system-based problem, not just an individual practice problem
- Prompt you to continually evaluate the risks involved in medication use in your everyday practice
- Stimulate professional practice changes that can reduce your risk of making a medication error
- Promote interdisciplinary teamwork among nurses and other healthcare providers to make system changes that will reduce the risk of harmful medication errors
- Provide you with drug safety information specific to high-risk patients, processes, and medications that have the greatest chance of causing harm if an error occurs

Every error is potentially tragic and costly in both human and economic terms for patients and healthcare providers alike. We hope this resource will provide you with an essential tool for learning more about medication errors and ways to lessen their potentially tragic consequences.

Hedy Cohen, RN, MSN
Judy Smetzer, RN, BSN
Nancy Tuohy, RN, MSN
Institute for Safe Medication Practices

INSTITUTE FOR SAFE MEDICATION PRACTICES (ISMP)

Who We Are
We are a nonprofit healthcare agency composed of pharmacists, nurses, and physicians. Founded in 1994, our organization is dedicated to learning about medication errors, understanding their system-based causes, and disseminating practical recommendations that can help healthcare providers, consumers, and the pharmaceutical industry prevent errors.

Who We Are Not
We are not a governmental, regulatory, licensing, inspecting, or accrediting agency. Although we work collaboratively with these types of agencies to influence medication safety, we do not set healthcare standards or require individual organizations to implement the recommendations we make.

How We Are Funded
As a nonprofit agency, we rely on charitable donations, unrestricted grants, subscriptions to our newsletters, and fees from our consulting and educational services. We are not funded by the pharmaceutical industry and do not accept advertising in any of our publications.

How We Learn about Medication Errors

Over 25 years ago, we started a voluntary error-reporting program to learn about medication errors that were happening across the nation. In January 1994, ISMP was chartered as a nonprofit agency to further this work. Today, the program, now called the USP-ISMP Medication Errors Reporting Program (MERP), continues to thrive. Each year, hundreds of healthcare professionals trust us enough to report errors to this program to help us learn about errors, understand their causes, and share the "lessons learned" with others. You too can report errors through our website (www.ismp.org), by e-mail (ismpinfo@ismp.org), or by calling 1-800-FAIL-SAF(E).

How We Keep Error Reports Confidential

While we share stories about medication errors in our publications and through other educational efforts, we have never disclosed the specific location of an event, the people involved, or the person who reported the error. When necessary, less important details about an error may be changed to ensure that inadvertent recognition of the error is not possible. In addition, if healthcare facilities seek our advice about a medication error or other medication safety issues, facility-specific recommendations are not disclosed publicly, even in a blinded manner.

How We Learn about Error-Reduction Strategies

Many years of analyzing medication error reports have enabled us to suggest credible error-reduction strategies. We are in constant contact with an advisory panel of practicing healthcare professionals, researchers, and experts in human factors and medication safety who collectively help us offer evidence-based and practical error-reduction strategies that work. In addition, our staff spends considerable time in healthcare facilities learning firsthand about innovative medication safety practices, so we can share these ideas with others.

What's Available on Our Website

We offer a wide variety of free educational materials and services on our website including:

- Special medication hazard alerts
- Searchable information on a wide variety of medication safety topics
- Answers to frequently asked questions about medication safety
- FDA patient safety videos
- Three Pathways for Medication Safety tools:
  - ▶ A model strategic plan for medication safety
  - ▶ Risk assessment tools and questions for clinicians

- ▸ Readiness assessment for bedside bar coding
- White papers on bar-coding technology and electronic prescribing
- A monitored message board to share questions, answers, and ideas

Other Ways We Can Help

Over the years, we have developed numerous publications, programs, and tools designed to help healthcare professionals prevent medication errors. For example, we:

- Publish three professional newsletters and one consumer newsletter (collectively reaching millions of readers)
- Conduct frequent educational programs, including teleconferences, on medication safety issues
- Offer posters, videos, patient brochures, books, and other drug safety tools
- Conduct on-site risk assessments of medication safety in healthcare facilities and respond to sentinel events

SYSTEM ELEMENTS

SEE ALSO

Key terms highlighted in **green** throughout
the text are defined in the **Glossary**.

Interdisciplinary Approach to Medication Use

As illustrated in the figure, the steps involved in getting the correct medications to patients can be diagrammed as one continuous complex process. Most would identify tasks I-L under the category of Administration/Patient Education as the nurse's primary role in medication use. However, nurses have a much broader role, often performing other tasks including:

- **Task A:** Obtaining and documenting the patient's medication history
- **Task D:** Transmitting the order to the pharmacy
- **Task E:** Verifying and transcribing the order on the medication administration record
- **Task M:** Documenting medication administration, and assessing the patient's response and notifying prescribers

In addition, nurses routinely interact with physicians, pharmacists, pharmacy technicians, and other clinicians to communicate information about the patient when they are:

- **Task B:** Deciding on therapy
- **Task F:** Evaluating the order
- **Task G:** Preparing the medication

These complex interactions between nurses and other clinicians and departments suggest that an *interdisciplinary approach* to medication use is needed to ensure patient safety. Nurses, physicians, pharmacists, unit secretaries, pharmacy technicians, respiratory therapists, and many other healthcare providers must work together as a team to reduce the risk of medication errors.

Sample Medication Process Diagram

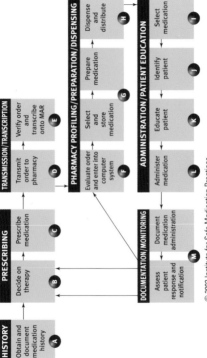

HISTORY
- **A** Obtain and document medication history

PRESCRIBING
- **B** Decide on therapy
- **C** Prescribe medication

TRANSMISSION/TRANSCRIPTION
- **D** Transmit order to pharmacy
- **E** Verify order and transcribe onto MAR

PHARMACY PROFILING/PREPARATION/DISPENSING
- **F** Evaluate order and enter into computer system
- **G** Select and store medication
- **G** Prepare medication
- **H** Dispense and distribute

ADMINISTRATION/PATIENT EDUCATION
- **I** Select medication
- **J** Identify patient
- **K** Educate patient
- **L** Administer medication

DOCUMENTATION/MONITORING
- **M** Document medication administration
- Assess patient response and notification

© 2002 Institute for Safe Medication Practices.

Adding a Systems-Based Approach to Medication Use[5]

An interdisciplinary approach to medication use is crucial because medication errors are caused by weaknesses that are common in systems *throughout* the organization. When a medication error occurs, these organization-wide system weaknesses are often related to:

- How you collect and communicate information about the patient
- How you collect and communicate information about medications
- How you interact with colleagues
- How you educate patients and staff about medications and error prevention
- How you manage the environment to promote performance and uninterrupted focus on critical tasks
- How you provide well-qualified and rested staff to carry out patient care and supportive healthcare functions
- How you learn about medication errors and their causes
- How you safeguard high-risk patients from harm

The table on page 6 provides details about the key system elements related to medication use. Weaknesses in these elements can be directly traced to the system-based causes of medication errors. The table also offers examples of selected safety strategies that are likely to reduce the risk of errors. The system-based causes of errors, as well as successful safety strategies, are best uncovered through interdisciplinary efforts.

The key system elements can be used to evaluate medication use in two ways—proactively (before an error occurs) and retrospectively (after an error occurs). For example, a new infusion pump, a new medication, or even parts of an existing process could be examined proactively to identify the risk of making errors, so that action can be taken to prevent the chance of serious patient harm. Most often, a process called **failure mode and effects analysis (FMEA)** is used to help uncover these risks. As part of this process, the key system elements can be used to prompt discussion about the possible causes of error. Retrospectively, a root cause analysis (RCA) is often used to determine causative factors. Again, the key system elements can be used to identify breakdowns in the system that led to the error.

System Analysis Reduces Blame

Unfortunately, when an error occurs, it is tempting to seek out individuals to blame. This is characteristic of a punitive environment. But analyzing errors in an *interdisciplinary systems-based* context helps you resist this temptation by looking broadly at the key system elements, not at individual people or departments, to determine the causes of errors. It does not remove individual accountability for medication safety, but instead expands accountability to all who could potentially influence the medication use process. In this way, accountability depends not on perfect job performance, but on identifying safety problems, implementing system-based solutions, and applying them to your practice.

ISMP Ten Key System Elements of Medication Use [5, 25A]

Weaknesses in these system elements can cause medication errors.

SYSTEM ELEMENT	EXAMPLES OF SAFETY PROBLEMS	EXAMPLES OF SAFETY STRATEGIES
Patient information (e.g., age, gender, diagnoses, pregnancy, allergies, height, weight, lab values, diagnostic study results, vital signs, ability to pay for prescriptions, patient identity) *Essential patient information is obtained, readily available in useful form, and considered when prescribing, dispensing, and administering medications.*	• Untimely access to lab studies • Failure to adjust doses for patients with hepatic or renal impairment • Patient allergies unknown • Teratogenic medication given to pregnant patient • Failure to notice significant respiratory depression in patients receiving IV opioids • Patient misidentified • Patient unable to pay for prescriptions • Patient weight unavailable for proper dosing	• Gain electronic access to lab values • Communicate patient allergies to pharmacy before medications are dispensed and administered • Obtain daily weights on high-risk patients and notify pharmacy of any changes • List allergies and diagnoses on order forms and MARs • Place allergy alert bracelets on patients • Use two unique identifiers (or bar coding) to confirm patient identity • Take MARs to the bedside during administration • Require special monitoring for high-risk patients (obesity, asthma, sleep apnea) receiving IV opioids • Assess patient's ability to pay for prescriptions, and refer to case management/social services if problems uncovered

6

Drug information (e.g., maximum dose, typical dose, route, precautions, contraindications, special warnings, drug interactions, cross allergies)	• Incomplete information about the patient's "home" medications • Knowledge deficit leading to administration of the wrong dose or use of the wrong route • Nurses unaware of special precautions or special monitoring needed with medication • Computer warnings about unsafe doses overlooked/ignored • Serious drug interaction unknown/overlooked	• Provide up-to-date, timely drug information (online and print) • Staff pharmacists in patient care units for consultation and education • Provide readily accessible dosing charts, protocols, guidelines, checklists for **high-alert medications** • Establish maximum doses for high-alert medications; list applicable doses on preprinted orders; build alerts in computers to warn staff if doses exceed safe limits • A pharmacist reviews all drug orders before administration (except emergency)
Essential drug information is readily available in useful form when ordering, dispensing, or administering medications.		
Communication (e.g., communication dynamics among colleagues, team dynamics, communication of drug orders)	• Failure to question orders or pursue safety concerns due to intimidation • Illegible handwritten orders • Error-prone presentation of medication orders on MARs	• Utilize electronic prescribing systems that connect to the pharmacy computer and electronic MAR • Use carefully designed standard preprinted orders • Prohibit error-prone abbreviations, symbols, and dose expressions on orders, MARs, labels, etc.

continued

SYSTEM ELEMENT	EXAMPLES OF SAFETY PROBLEMS	EXAMPLES OF SAFETY STRATEGIES
Methods of communicating drug orders and other drug information are standardized and automated to minimize the risk for error.	• Incomplete medication orders (missing dose or route, orders to "resume same medications" upon transfer, or "take home medications" upon admission) • Abbreviations misunderstood (e.g., U misread as a zero) • Misheard verbal orders • Failure to transmit all orders to pharmacy	• Discourage verbal orders except in emergencies and prohibit for high-risk medications and antineoplastics • Document verbal orders on the chart when accepted, and read back the orders to confirm • Require complete orders (not "resume" orders) upon admission, transfer, and discharge • Establish a procedure that specifies the steps practitioners should take when there is disagreement about the safety of an order • Send all orders to the pharmacy, even if the medication prescribed is available on the unit, or the order is for a treatment but does not contain the name of a medication—it may indicate a clinical change for the pharmacy profile
Drug names, labels, and packages *Readable labels that clearly identify drugs and doses are*	• Product misidentification due to look-alike drug labels and packages, or look-/sound-alike drug names • Confusing or ambiguous labels	• Dispense medications in labeled, unit-dose form • Label all syringes with name and strength of drug • Keep oral medications in original packaging until administered at the bedside

continued

on all medication containers, and labels remain up to the point of administration. *Strategies are undertaken to minimize the possibility of errors with products that have similar or confusing labels/packages or names.*	• Unlabeled medications/syringes • Unlabeled solutions/syringes on the sterile field • Poorly positioned labels that obscure vital information • Doses dispensed in bulk supplies without patient-specific labels • Mislabeled medications	• Store drugs with look-alike names/packages in separate areas or drawers of automated dispensing cabinets • Use warning labels to alert staff to unusual strengths, special precautions • Ensure pharmacy labels are easy for nurses to read and understand • Require prescribers to include the indication for *prn* medications to differentiate them from drugs with look-alike names
Drug standardization, storage, and distribution (e.g., storage of unit stock medications and pharmacy-dispensed medications, preparation of IV medications, use of standard concentrations, pharmacy delivery services)	• Multiple concentrations of IV solutions leading to potential use of the wrong concentration • Nurse preparation of IV solutions • Failure to dilute concentrated medications and electrolytes properly before administration • Selection of the wrong drug or dose caused by unsafe storage of medications on patient care units	• Standardize concentrations of insulin, heparin, morphine, and vasopressor drips (adult and pediatric) to a single concentration for each drug • Use commercially available premixed IV solutions whenever possible • Limit nurse preparation of IV solutions to emergency situations only • Dispense medications from the pharmacy according to realistic timeframes for stat, urgent, and routine medications

SYSTEM ELEMENT	EXAMPLES OF SAFETY PROBLEMS	EXAMPLES OF SAFETY STRATEGIES
IV solutions, drug concentrations, and administration times are standard when possible. *Medications are provided to patient care units in a safe and secure manner and available for administration within a timeframe that meets essential patient needs.* *Unit-based floor stock is restricted.*	• Hazardous chemicals, fixatives, and developers stored with medications, leading to mix-ups • Missing medications due to problems with pharmacy distribution or nursing transmission of orders • Nonstandard medication administration times • Delay in therapy due to untimely delivery of new medications or failure of nursing transmission of order • Unsafe nursing access to pharmacy after hours	• Store high-alert medications in pharmacy until needed for a specific patient or secure and restrict access if available on unit • Remove concentrated forms of electrolytes from patient care units • Provide all stock medications in unit-dose form (no bulk supplies) • Remove discontinued medications from the unit in a timely manner; do not borrow medications from patient supplies • Prohibit nursing access to the pharmacy after hours; establish a night cabinet with a restricted supply of medications for use when pharmacy closed
Medication delivery devices (e.g., infusion pumps, implantable pumps, oral and parenteral syringes, glucose monitors)	• Pump programming errors • Accidental administration of an oral solution by the IV route • Rapid free-flow of solution when tubing removed from pump	• Examine new devices for the potential for errors before purchase and use (see **Assessing Risk** for more information) • Limit the variety of infusion pumps to promote user proficiency

continued

The potential for human error is mitigated through careful procurement, maintenance, use, and standardization of devices used to prepare and deliver medications.	• Failure to notice incorrect default setting on pump, leading to dosing errors • Unfamiliarity with medication delivery devices, leading to misuse • Line mix-ups (connecting an IV solution to an epidural line) • Insufficient supply of infusion pumps to meet patient needs • End-users (often nurses) not involved in purchase decisions regarding medication delivery devices	• Prohibit the use of infusion pumps without free-flow protection • Educate staff adequately about use of new devices and ensure competency before independent use • Require one nurse to set up a pump and another to **independently double check** the order, solution, settings, line attachment, and patient before infusing IV solutions that contain high-alert medications • Label the distal ends of all tubing if patients are receiving solutions via multiple routes (IV, arterial, enteral, epidural, bladder installation) • Use specially-designed oral syringes to administer oral solutions to prevent inadvertent connection to an IV port • Purchase and use "smart" pumps that offer technology to intercept and prevent wrong dose/infusion rate errors

ISMP Ten Key System Elements of Medication Use (continued)

SYSTEM ELEMENT	EXAMPLES OF SAFETY PROBLEMS	EXAMPLES OF SAFETY STRATEGIES
Environmental factors and staffing patterns (e.g., physical surroundings, physical health of staff, organization of unit, lighting, noise, foot traffic, storage, ergonomics, work overload, adequate staffing, safe work schedules)	• Drug mix-ups due to lack of space or cluttered workspaces • Drug mix-ups due to overfilled and disorganized storage in refrigerators • Misinterpreted verbal/telephone orders due to noise and distractions • Errors in preparation or drug mix-ups due to poorly lighted workspaces and drug storage cabinets	• Ensure adequate space, storage, and lighting in stock medication areas, including automated dispensing cabinets • Provide workspaces that are free of distractions for transcription of medication orders • Arrange areas for IV and oral dose preparation that are isolated from noise, foot traffic, or distractions • Make computers and patient monitors adjustable for staff comfort and safety when using
Medications are prescribed, transcribed, prepared, and administered in an environment with adequate space and lighting to allow complete focus on medication use.	• Interruptions during medication preparation or administration causing mental slips and other errors • Inadequate staffing patterns leading to task overload and rushed procedures • Staff member fatigue causing impaired judgment and flawed performance • Mental overload and error potential due to inadequate breaks	• Purchase refrigerators that are of adequate size for organized storage of medication • Establish a realistic staffing plan to safely provide care to patients during staff illnesses, vacations, and patient acuity fluctuations • Schedule adequate staffing to allow for meals/breaks
The complement of qualified, well-rested practitioners matches the clinical workload		• Manage and monitor individual staff schedules to allow adequate rest between shifts, and to prohibit shifts longer than 12 hours

without compromising patient safety.		• Minimize the use of transient agency staff • Communicate plans for new services to all involved staff, and carefully consider the resources necessary so that additional work volume will be met without compromising patient safety
Staff competency and education (e.g., orientation, in-service education, certifications, annual competencies, skills labs, simulation of events, off-site education) *Practitioners receive sufficient orientation to medication use and undergo baseline and annual competency evaluation of knowledge and skills related to safe medication practices.*	• Lack of staffing contingency plans to cover illness and vacations • Human resources required for new services not fully considered • Delays and errors due to misunderstanding between nursing and pharmacy stemming from lack of knowledge of each discipline's practice patterns and environments • Inappropriate medication doses or errors in patient assessment and monitoring due to lack of knowledge about particular patient populations • Errors related to task overload and rushed procedures for those with added responsibility of training new staff	• Organize all orientation schedules according to individual learning needs and assessments • Arrange staffing so that preceptors have reduced workload to avoid overload of normal duties • Require new nurses to spend time in the pharmacy to become familiar with drug dispensing processes • Require new pharmacists to spend time on patient care units to become familiar with drug administration processes • Provide staff education about new medications before they are used • Require pharmacy to affix special alerts or provide other important information about non-formulary drugs when dispensing these medications

continued

SYSTEM ELEMENT	EXAMPLES OF SAFETY PROBLEMS	EXAMPLES OF SAFETY STRATEGIES
Practitioners involved in medication use are provided with ongoing education about medication error prevention and the safe use of drugs that have the greatest potential to cause harm if misused.	• Medication errors by new or reassigned ("floated") nurses who are required to perform unfamiliar tasks or administer unfamiliar medications without proper orientation, education, or supervision • Errors with new medications administered to patients without full knowledge of the preparation, dose, route, action, or anticipated effects • Errors (including near misses) are often unreported, and knowledge about the causes of errors and their prevention is lost	• Ensure that reassignment to other units ("floating") is not permitted until staff have undergone orientation and recent competency verification • Provide staff with ongoing education about medication errors that have occurred within the organization and in other organizations, as well as strategies to prevent these errors • Create job descriptions and performance evaluations that include specific accountability standards for patient/medication safety and that do not include the absence of errors or a numeric error threshold • Provide staff with the necessary support and time to attend internal and external education programs related to medication use and error prevention
Patient education (e.g., drug information sheets, dosing schedules for complex medication regimens, discharge instructions, tips to	• Patients might feel uncomfortable reminding staff to verify their identity • Patients might be reluctant to ask questions about the medications they are receiving	• Teach patients how to actively participate in proper identification before accepting medication or undergoing procedures • Provide patients/families with the brand and generic name of the medication, the general purpose, the

continued

avoid errors, consumer representation in drug safety efforts) *Patients are included as active partners in their care through education about their medications and ways to avert errors.*	• Patients might not understand information given to them verbally because of medical jargon or other language barriers • Low health literacy or poor reading skills might prevent patients from understanding printed information or directions for using medications • Patients often lack resources for questions about drug therapy after discharge • Patients might not remember all the medications and doses they are taking, increasing the risk of errors when prescribing medications upon admission • Patients lack information about the causes of medication errors and how to prevent them	prescribed dose, and important side effects for each medication administered • Consult a pharmacist for assistance, especially if patients are, or will be, taking more than five medications at home • Encourage patients to ask questions about their drug therapy • Fully investigate and resolve all patient questions about drug therapy before drug administration • Provide patients with written materials that use lay terminology (8th grade reading level or lower) for **high-alert medications** prescribed at discharge • Instruct patients on when and whom to call for concerns about their drug therapy after discharge • Encourage patients to keep a current written record of all their prescription and over-the-counter medications, herbal products, and vitamins, and to show the list to healthcare providers during each visit • Help patients who take multiple medications create a MAR for home use

15

SYSTEM ELEMENT	EXAMPLES OF SAFETY PROBLEMS	EXAMPLES OF SAFETY STRATEGIES
Quality process and risk management (e.g., culture, leadership, error reporting, safety strategies, safety redundancies) *A non-punitive, systems-based approach to error reduction is in place and supported by management, senior administration, and the Board of Trustees.* *Practitioners are stimulated to detect and report errors, and interdisciplinary teams regularly analyze errors that have occurred within the organization and in other*	• Lack of leadership and budgetary support for medication safety • Disincentives (shame, blame, fear of disciplinary action, documentation of errors in personnel files) encourage underreporting of errors • Culture of secrecy and blame prevents disclosure of errors to patients/families • Inaccurate error rates determined using error reports, with a counterproductive goal of reducing the number of error reports • Ineffective error prevention strategies focused on individual performance improvement, rather than system improvements • Lack of understanding of medication administration as a system and ways to safeguard the system as a whole	• Clearly articulate patient/medication safety in the organization's mission/vision/values statements • Educate mid-level mangers to effectively evaluate competency and handle difficult behavior without allowing presence/absence of errors to be a factor • Promote a culture where human error is anticipated and accountability for safety is shared among organizational leaders and staff without blame • Promote and reward reporting of errors and hazardous conditions that could lead to errors; expect a sustained, not reduced, error-reporting rate • Disclose errors that reach a patient • Include discussions about errors and their prevention in all staff meetings as a standing agenda item • Convene an interdisciplinary team to routinely review errors and other safety data to identify system-based causes and facilitate implementation of system-based enhancements

organizations for the purpose of redesigning systems to best support safe practitioner performance. Simple redundancies that support a system of independent double checks or an automated verification process are used for vulnerable parts of the medication use process to detect and correct errors before they reach patients.	• Lack of automated or manual double checks in place for critical steps in the medication use process • Failed manual double checks, often because they are not performed independently • Misplacement/misuse of double checks in place of system enhancements that would prevent errors	• Invite patient/community representatives to participate in medication safety discussions to solicit their input • Disseminate ongoing information throughout the organization about errors and safety strategies • Recalculate all doses for antineoplastics and pediatric medications to verify the prescriber's order • Perform an independent double check (manual or automated) to verify the drug, dose, concentration, infusion rate, patient, route, and line attachment before administering selected high-alert medications such as IV insulin, IV antineoplastics, and IV opioids (including PCA) • Employ bar coding technology during drug administration

MAR or **MARs**, medication administration record(s).

HIGH-ALERT DRUGS

Key terms highlighted in **green** throughout
the text are defined in the **Glossary**.

DEFINING HIGH-ALERT DRUGS[25]

High-alert drugs bear a heightened risk of causing significant patient harm when they are used in error. Mistakes may or may not be more common with these drugs, but the consequences of an error with these medications are more devastating to patients. Knowing which medications are considered high-alert will remind you to employ additional safety strategies when preparing and administering these drugs.

These medications were selected through careful review of voluntarily submitted reports of medication errors that have actually caused significant patient harm. Your organization may add to this list according to your experiences.

Specific High-Alert Medications[14]
- amiodarone, IV
- colchicine, injection
- dextrose, hypertonic (20% or greater)
- heparin, low molecular weight, injection
- heparin, unfractionated, IV
- insulin, subcutaneous and IV
- lidocaine, IV
- magnesium sulfate injection
- methotrexate, oral nononcologic use (arthritis)
- nesiritide
- potassium chloride concentrate for injection
- potassium phosphates for injection
- sodium chloride injection (hypertonic, i.e., greater than 0.9% concentration)
- sodium nitroprusside for injection
- warfarin

High-Alert Medications by Class/Category/Type[14]

MEDICATION CLASS/CATEGORY/TYPE	EXAMPLES OR DESCRIPTION
Adrenergic agonists, IV	epinephrine, isoproterenol, norepinephrine
Adrenergic antagonists, IV	propranolol
General anesthetics, inhalation or IV	propofol
Antineoplastic agents, parenteral and oral	cyclophosphamide, methotrexate
Cardioplegic solutions	various formulations
Dextrose, hypertonic, 20% or greater	
Dialysis solutions	peritoneal dialysis or hemodialysis
Epidural and intrathecal medications	opioid, anesthetic
Glycoprotein IIb/IIIa inhibitors	eptifibatide
Hypoglycemics, oral and insulins	glyburide, rosiglitazone
Inotropic drugs, IV	digoxin, milrinone
Liposomal drug forms	liposomal amphotericin B
Conscious sedation agents, IV	midazolam
Conscious sedation agents, oral, for children	chloral hydrate, midazolam
Neuromuscular blocking agents	succinylcholine
Opioids, IV and oral, including liquid concentrates and immediate- and sustained-release forms	morphine, fentanyl, hydromorphone
Radiocontrast agents, IV	diatrizoate, iothalamate
Thrombolytics/fibrinolytics, IV	tenecteplase
Total parenteral nutrition solutions	

HIGH-ALERT DRUG SAFETY[5]

There are three primary goals for safeguarding **high-alert medications** including:

- Reduce or eliminate the possibility of an error
- Make errors visible before they reach the patient
- Minimize the consequences of an error if it does reach the patient

Reduce or Eliminate Errors

The best way to safeguard high-alert medications is to *prevent* errors in the first place. This requires system changes that eliminate all possibility of an error. For example, if you always draw liquid oral medications into a specially designed oral syringe, another healthcare provider cannot possibly pick up the syringe and, believing it is a different medication, administer it IV. Oral syringes cannot be connected to an IV port, which eliminates the possibility of this error. Other safety strategies can also be employed to *reduce the risk of an error* or make it less likely to happen. Examples include educating staff or using protocols to guide drug administration. However, these types of safety strategies may still allow for the possibility of an occasional error.

Make Errors Visible

Because it is unlikely that all errors with high-alert drugs will be prevented, the second safeguard is to make errors visible when they do occur. Examples include having two nurses independently recalculate the patient's prescribed dose of cancer chemotherapy, or using a bar coding system to verify that the correct drug, dose, and patient have been selected.

Minimize the Consequences of an Error

Systems must be designed to reduce the risk of harm to the patient in the event that an error with a high-alert medication occurs. Frequent or special monitoring may be needed so that the effects of an error can be detected quickly and antidotes can be given.

KEY SAFETY PRINCIPLES

Experts in the field of human performance have established some key safety principles that can be incorporated into healthcare processes to safeguard high-alert medications. These principles are meant to compensate for our inability to perform flawlessly. They help us overcome limitations such as the unpredictable and unintentional mental states—such as forgetfulness, momentary inattention, preoccupation, and distractibility—that sometimes lead to errors. By making automatic tasks a little less automatic, or by removing complex steps in a process, the risk of an error can be reduced.

Key Safety Principles for Safeguarding High-Alert Medications [5A]

KEY PRINCIPLES	DESCRIPTION		EXAMPLES
Simplify	Reduce the number of steps, hand-offs, and options without eliminating crucial redundancies		• Use commercially available premixed solutions instead of preparing IV solutions
			• Consult dosing charts instead of manually calculating infusion rates
	Steps in process*	**Error probability**	• Limit drug choice to a single concentration
	1	1%	• Dispense oral and parenteral medications in the most ready-to-use form (unit-dose packages)
	25	22%	• Transmit orders to pharmacy electronically (via scanning or computerized prescribing)
	50	39%	
	100	63%	
	* each step is 99% reliable		
Externalize or centralize error-prone processes	Transfer error-prone tasks to an external site or centralized area to ensure that they are completed in a distraction-free environment by those who have expertise, and that appropriate quality control steps (e.g., sterility measures, double checks) are carried out		• Use commercially prepared products
			• Have pharmacy prepare all IV solutions under sterile conditions
			• Use a specialized external service to prepare complicated solutions such as TPN, dialysate, cardioplegic solutions

Differentiate items	Modify the packages and labels of medications to help distinguish them from other medications with look-alike packages or look-alike names	• Affix auxiliary labels to make medications look different or to call attention to important information • Use color to draw out warning labels • Use a pen or marker to circle important information on medication labels or MARs • Purchase look-alike medications from different manufacturers to maximize label differences • Use tactile clues such as placing rubber bands on the vial of long-acting insulin to differentiate it from short-acting insulin • Use **tall man lettering** on labels and MARs to call out differences in look-alike drug names (e.g., HumaLOG and HumuLIN)
Standardize	Create clinically sound, uniform models of care that should be adhered to when carrying out various functions related to medication use in order to reduce variation and complexity in the processes	• Use carefully designed preprinted order sets, protocols, and clinical pathways to standardize high-risk processes and the administration of **high-alert medications** • Gain consensus among physicians who treat similar disease states and establish one standard order set for each standardized care process • Establish a controlled vocabulary in which the use of error-prone abbreviations, symbols, and dose expressions is prohibited

continued

Key Safety Principles for Safeguarding High-Alert Medications (continued)

KEY PRINCIPLES	DESCRIPTION	EXAMPLES
		• Standardize the sliding scale used to prescribe insulin coverage and design/use a preprinted order form
		• Standardize to a single concentration and container size whenever possible for all high-alert medications
Redundancies	Implement duplicate steps in a process to force additional checks in the system; employ more than one qualified and trained staff member to carry out specialized processes to ensure ability to perform critical functions	• Perform an independent double check* for critical steps in the medication use process
		• Employ automated check systems such as bar coding or use "smart" IV infusion pumps that alarm when a drug infusion rate exceeds safe limits
		• Ask patients about drug allergies each time drug is administered
		• Ask prescribers to review handwritten orders with a nurse before leaving the unit
		• Cross-train selected staff to perform critical medication use functions and maintain proficiency through ongoing experiences
Reminders	Provide additional alerts or warnings to make important information highly visible so it is remembered when	• Affix auxiliary labels to medications or add highlighted notes to MARs to remind staff about important functions (e.g., check for pregnancy or cross allergies)

	carrying out medication use processes	• Label IV lines • Use checklists for complex processes • Build reminders for special monitoring into order sets or protocols • Set visual and audible alarms on equipment • Build reminders into screens on automated dispensing cabinets (e.g., measure dose using dropper provided)
Improve access to information	Use active, not passive, means of providing staff and patients with necessary information at the exact time when needed while performing critical tasks related to medication use	• Provide current drug reference texts or an electronic database at the point of drug administration for easy access when needed • Provide easy access to quick drug reference tables at the point of drug administration • Increase visibility of pharmacists in patient care units for immediate consultation when needed • Include the medical librarian on patient rounds to follow through with dissemination of patient education materials • Use computer order entry systems that merge patient and drug information, thus providing immediate warnings if unsafe orders are entered

continued

Key Safety Principles for Safeguarding High-Alert Medications (continued)

KEY PRINCIPLES	DESCRIPTION	EXAMPLES
Limit access or use	Use constraints to restrict access to certain medications or error-prone conditions; require special education or conditions for prescribing, dispensing, or administering a particular drug; require special authorization for participation in certain critical tasks related to medication use	• Prohibit nursing (or other non-pharmacy staff) access to the pharmacy after it is closed • Carefully select the drugs, concentrations, and quantities available in unit stock • Remove all concentrated electrolytes from patient care areas • Store neuromuscular blocking agents in a separate container to limit access • Use automatic stop orders to limit the dose or duration of medication therapy • Require special education/credentialing for use of certain **high-alert medications** (e.g., antineoplastics, conscious sedation, PCA) • Establish parameters to change IV therapy to oral therapy as soon as possible • Minimize the variety of medication choices and dose ranges on preprinted order forms

Forcing functions and fail-safes	Employ procedures or equipment design features that will: • prevent something from happening until certain conditions are met (forcing function) OR • prevent malfunctioning or unintentional operation by reverting back to a predetermined safe state if a failure occurs (fail-safe)	• Use oral syringes that cannot be connected to IV tubing ports • Use medication ordering programs that cannot process an order unless key information, such as allergies and weight, has been entered • Use automated dispensing cabinets that require pharmacy review of medication orders before access to the drug is provided • Use infusion pumps with an automatic clamping mechanism to prevent free-flow if the tubing is removed from the pump • Use epidural tubing without ports • Use PCA pumps with default settings of zero, or the highest possible concentration for the opioids used
Patient monitoring	Assess the effects of medication through a constant feedback loop of predetermined patient parameters evaluated at set intervals	• Prospectively establish parameters (e.g., vital signs, quality of respirations, lab tests, observation, neurological signs) for monitoring patients who are receiving high-alert medications • Concurrently monitor patients who are receiving high-alert drugs for medication effects • Retrospectively monitor the effects of medications on groups of patients via chart audits aimed at detecting untoward drug events (e.g., insulin-induced hypoglycemia, heparin/warfarin-induced bleeding, chemotherapy-induced leukopenia, use of an antidote to reverse oversedation)

continued

Key Safety Principles for Safeguarding High-Alert Medications (continued)

KEY PRINCIPLES	DESCRIPTION	EXAMPLES
Failure mode and effects analysis (FMEA)**	Convene a team to proactively identify the ways that a process or medication-related equipment can fail, why it might fail, how it might affect patients, and how it can be made safer	• Perform a **FMEA** on a new high-alert medication before allowing its use • Perform a FMEA on a new infusion pump being considered for purchase • Perform a FMEA on a high-risk process or sub-process related to medication use (e.g., order transcription, selecting medications from automated dispensing cabinets, patient-controlled analgesia, administration of antineoplastics)

MAR or **MARs**, medication administration record(s).

*See guidelines for performing a manual independent double check on page 42.
Additional information on FMEA can be found in **Assessing Risk.

Strategies to safely use antineoplastics, insulin, heparin, warfarin, and concentrated electrolytes follow. Ways to measure the effectiveness of implementing the suggested strategies are also included. Collecting data on these measures, both before and after implementation, will let you know if the strategies resulted in improvement or if more needs to be done to protect your patients from harm.

Antineoplastics

KEY PRINCIPLES	SAFETY STRATEGIES	EVALUATION CRITERIA
Standardize and simplify	• Use carefully designed preprinted order forms or computer order sets for all antineoplastics • Specify single or daily doses • Include both the mg/m² (or AUC) dose and the calculated dose • Avoid all abbreviations, drug name stems, and acronyms • Require documentation of the rationale for dose adjustments • Prohibit verbal orders for antineoplastics	• Number of antineoplastics orders found during the order entry process that fail to comply with standardized order communication requirements per total number of antineoplastics orders *(pharmacy checkpoint)*
Improve access to drug information	• Establish dose limits for maximum single dose, daily dose, course dose, and lifetime dose • Build alerts into information systems to warn staff about exceeding maximum safe doses for antineoplastics • Approve all unusual doses through peer review before dispensing or administering antineoplastics • Make protocols/information about commonly used regimens available in the pharmacy/patient care units	• Number of antineoplastics doses found during the order entry process that exceed established maximum doses per total number of antineoplastics orders *(pharmacy checkpoint)*

	• Increase visibility of pharmacists in patient care areas where antineoplastics are administered • Maintain ongoing patient profiles for all patients who receive antineoplastics	
Improve access to patient information	• Establish a system to communicate height, weight, pertinent laboratory values, and allergies to the pharmacy where antineoplastics are prepared and dispensed	• Number of pharmacy computer profiles without patient height, weight, and allergies per all oncology patient profiles *(pharmacy checkpoint)*
Redundancies	• Establish a system of **independent double checks** in the pharmacy for dose calculation and antineoplastics preparation • Establish a system of independent double checks on patient care units to verify the drug, dose (including calculations), infusion pump settings, connection to correct line and pump, and correct patient before administering antineoplastics	• Number of calculation errors identified during independent double check process per total number of antineoplastics orders *(nursing and pharmacy checkpoints)*
Limit access or use	• Allow only oncology-certified nurses to administer antineoplastics • Allow only specially trained pharmacists or technicians to prepare, check, and dispense antineoplastics • Allow only certified oncologists to prescribe antineoplastics	• Number of oncology-certified nurses per total number of nurses providing care to oncology patients *(nursing checkpoint)*

Insulin

KEY PRINCIPLES	SAFETY STRATEGIES	EVALUATION CRITERIA
Standardize and simplify	• Use standardized sliding scales for subcutaneous insulin coverage • Use dosing/infusion rate charts for IV infusions • Use preprinted order forms for insulin infusions • Prohibit the abbreviation u for units • Prohibit verbal orders for insulin except in true emergency situations • Transcribe, then read back verbal orders and express the dose using single-digit numbers (one-five, not fifteen) • Standardize concentrations of insulin for IV infusions	• Number of times the abbreviation u appears with insulin orders per total number of insulin orders *(chart audit)* • Number of orders for insulin coverage not using standardized sliding scale per total number of insulin coverage orders *(nursing or pharmacy checkpoints)* • Number of verbal orders for insulin per total number of insulin orders *(chart audit)* • Number of orders for IV infusions with non-standard concentration of insulin per total number of orders for IV insulin infusions *(pharmacy checkpoint)* • Incidence of blood sugars less than 70 mg/dL per total number of patients receiving insulin *(chart audit or lab value screening)*

Improve access to patient information	• Perform blood glucose monitoring on patient care units and communicate in a standardized mode • Use blood glucose flow sheets and maintain them with the patient's MAR	• Incidence of blood sugars greater than 300 mg/dL per total number patients receiving insulin *(chart audit or lab value screening)* • Incidence of administering 50% dextrose or orange juice for symptoms of hypoglycemia per total number of patients receiving insulin *(chart audit, lab value screening, or computer trigger)* • Number of errors identified during independent double check processes per total number of patients receiving insulin *(nursing and pharmacy checkpoints)*
Redundancies	• Establish a system of independent double checks in patient care areas before administration of subcutaneous insulin • Establish a system of independent double checks on patient care units to verify the drug, dose, concentration, infusion pump settings, connection to correct line and pump, and correct patient before administering IV insulin • Require a pharmacist to independently check all insulin added to TPN solutions	
Limit or restrict drug access	• Separate look-alike products when using or storing • Keep insulin vials off counters and medication carts	

Heparin and Warfarin

KEY PRINCIPLES	SAFETY STRATEGIES	EVALUATION CRITERIA
Standardize and simplify	• Implement a weight-based heparin protocol • Use standardized preprinted orders for heparin infusions • Prohibit the abbreviation u for units • When necessary, use fractions, rather than decimal points when ordering warfarin doses (e.g., 2 1/2 mg, not 2.5 mg) • Use standard concentrations of premixed heparin solutions • Provide patient care units with prefilled heparin syringes for flushing lines • Provide patient care units with prefilled low-molecular-weight heparin syringes	• Number of heparin/warfarin orders found during the order entry process that fail to comply with standardized order communication requirements per total number of heparin/warfarin orders *(chart audit)* • Compliance with weight-based heparin protocol per total number of patients receiving IV heparin infusions *(chart audit)*
Use warnings and reminders	• Apply warning labels to distinguish low-molecular-weight heparin syringes from heparin flush syringes • Build alerts into information systems to warn against duplicate anticoagulant therapies • Build alerts into information systems to alert providers to drug interactions with warfarin	

Improve access to drug information	• Using drug interaction software, screen all orders for warfarin before dispensing or administering the drug • Use dosing/infusion charts for heparin infusions	• Number of drug interactions detected per total number of warfarin drug orders *(pharmacy computer printout)* • Number of pharmacist recommendations accepted per total number of drug interactions reported to prescribers *(pharmacy checkpoint)*
Improve access to patient information	• Call results of all aPTTs to the patient care unit within 2 hours, or monitor aPTTs at the bedside • Link information systems to communicate between prescribers, nursing, pharmacy, and laboratory • Place alert on patient chart if patient received thrombolytics (including low-molecular-weight heparin) or is changed from one anticoagulant (low-molecular-weight heparin, antiplatelet agent) to another • Communicate to pharmacy all doses of thrombolytics administered to the patient in the ED (including low-molecular-weight heparin) if patient admitted to the hospital	• Incidence of aPTT greater than 100 seconds per total number of patients receiving heparin *(chart audit or lab value screening)* • Incidence of INRs greater than 5 per total number of patients receiving warfarin *(chart audit or lab value screening)*

continued

Heparin and Warfarin (continued)

KEY PRINCIPLES	SAFETY STRATEGIES	EVALUATION CRITERIA
	• Use anticoagulation flow sheets and maintain them with the patient's MAR • Have anticoagulation flow sheets (listing drug orders, lab values, and other pertinent information) accompany the patient through transitions of care from the hospital to other skilled care or home • Establish a warfarin dosing service or "clinic" for inpatients and outpatients	• Incidence of administering vitamin K or FFP per total number of patients receiving heparin *(chart audit, lab value screening, or computer trigger)* • Episodes of bleeding per total patients receiving heparin or warfarin *(chart audit, computer or lab trigger)*
Redundancies	• Establish a system of independent double checks on patient care units to verify the drug, dose, concentration, infusion pump settings, connection to correct line and pump, and correct patient before administering IV heparin	• Number of errors identified during independent double check processes per total number of patients receiving IV heparin *(nursing and pharmacy checkpoints)*

FFP, fresh frozen plasma.

Concentrated Electrolytes (potassium chloride, potassium phosphate, sodium chloride)		
KEY PRINCIPLES	**SAFETY STRATEGIES**	**EVALUATION CRITERIA**
Standardize and simplify	• Establish protocols or guidelines for electrolyte replacement and use preprinted order forms • Standardize the terminology and dose expressions for ordering electrolytes • Standardize the method of ordering neonatal electrolyte solutions (e.g., by total electrolyte composition per volume for a 24-hour solution) • Require drugs with multiple electrolyte composition to be ordered as the dose for each component (potassium phosphate, sodium phosphate, etc.) • Require prescribers to include the mEq/kg (or mmol/kg, mg/kg, etc.) dose along with the calculated dose on all orders for neonatal and pediatric electrolytes • Establish parameters for concentrations and infusion rates of electrolyte solutions to be administered via infusion pumps	• Number of electrolyte orders found during the order entry process that fail to comply with standardized order communication requirements per total number of orders for electrolyte replacement *(pharmacy checkpoint)*

continued

Concentrated Electrolytes (potassium chloride, potassium phosphate, sodium chloride) (continued)

KEY PRINCIPLES	SAFETY STRATEGIES	EVALUATION CRITERIA
Use warnings and reminders	• Build alerts into the order entry computer systems to warn staff about exceeding maximum safe doses for electrolytes (including drugs with electrolyte ingredients such as penicillin G potassium and sodium) • Add warning label to alert staff to differing concentrations	• Number of electrolyte doses found during order entry process that exceed established maximum doses per total number of electrolyte replacement orders *(pharmacy checkpoint)*
Patient monitoring	• Include patient monitoring parameters (serum drug levels, EKG, etc.) on preprinted orders for electrolyte replacement therapy	• Incidence of patients with low or high electrolyte levels after receiving replacement therapy per total number of patients receiving electrolyte replacement therapy *(chart audit or lab value screening)* • Incidence of administering an antidote (Kayexalate, etc.) for excessive electrolyte levels per total number of patients receiving electrolyte replacement therapy *(chart audit; lab value screening, or computer trigger)*

Limit or restrict drug access	• Eliminate (or restrict) unit stock of concentrated electrolytes in patient care areas • Have pharmacy prepare all IVs containing electrolytes or provide solutions in commercially available premixed containers	
Redundancies	• Establish a system of nursing and pharmacy **independent double checks** for all dose calculations • Establish a system of independent double checks on patient care units to verify the drug, dose, concentration, infusion pump settings, connection to correct line and pump, and correct patient before administering adult IV concentrated electrolytes or any neonatal or pediatric electrolyte solution	• Number of errors identified during independent double check processes per total number of patients receiving IV concentrated electrolytes and pediatric electrolyte solutions *(nursing and pharmacy checkpoints)*

▮ INDEPENDENT DOUBLE CHECK [23, 25] ▮

A manual **independent double check** requires *two* individuals, preferably two licensed healthcare practitioners, to *separately* check each component of the work process. For example, one healthcare practitioner calculates a medication dose for a specific patient, and the second healthcare practitioner *independently* performs the same calculation and matches the results for verification.

Two people are unlikely to make the same mistake if they perform the same task *independently*. However, if two people work together performing the same task, both could be drawn into the conditions at that moment that lead to an error, making the **redundancy** in the process ineffective. So just asking another person to "look over my math" is not an effective way to carry out a double check.

Studies show that an independent double check is at least 95% effective. But there may be conditions in the environment that lead *both* practitioners to make the same mistake. For example, both practitioners may misread a confusing drug label or a poorly legible handwritten order, even if the task is performed independently. This is why an independent double check should never be used as the *only* safety strategy to safeguard a **high-alert medication**.

Key terms highlighted in **green** throughout
the text are defined in the **Glossary**.

LOOK- & SOUND-ALIKES

At one time or another, each of us has purchased the wrong product because of similarities between the item we intended to select and another item. Accidentally picking up a Pepsi rather than Diet Pepsi is a perfect example—the containers are similar in color, print, size, and shape, and both have Pepsi as part of the product name.

Similar mix-ups occur with medications that have look- or sound-alike names or packages, although the consequences are often much greater than those of selecting the wrong beverage. Unfortunately, with so many different medications on the market, striking similarities in drug names and packaging are rather common.

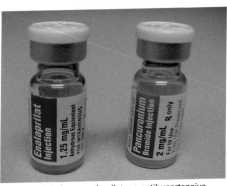

Look-alike labels on enalaprilat, an antihypertensive, and pancuronium, a neuromuscular blocking agent. Mix-ups could prove deadly, since pancuronium paralyzes the respiratory muscles, requiring mechanical ventilation.

Errors can occur when important information appears in an obscure position. The front of the Bentyl vial clearly states a concentration of 10 mg/mL. The vial actually contains 2 mL (20 mg of Bentyl), but this information is hidden on the back of the vial, along with an important precaution to administer the medication intramuscularly only.

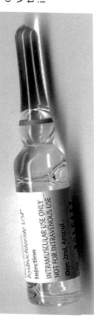

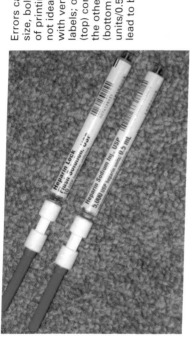

Errors can occur when size, bolding, and contrast of printing on labels are not ideal. Look-alike syringes with very small lettering on labels; one a heparin flush (top) containing 10 units/mL; the other a therapeutic dose (bottom) containing 5,000 units/0.5 mL. Mix-ups could lead to bleeding episodes.

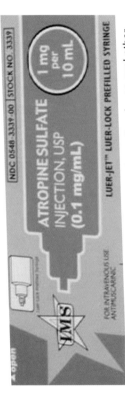

Errors can also occur when nonessential information, logos, and other special designs on the label distract from product identification. This highly stylized label design, depicting a star and a syringe, might distract from reading the label properly during an emergency.

Despite careful reading of labels, errors are often induced by familiarity with medications, coupled with the innate human tendency to perceive confirming evidence more readily than disconfirming evidence. This phenomenon, called *confirmation bias,* literally makes us see what is familiar, rather than what is actually there. As we gain experience, we develop a picture in our mind of what commonly used medications look like. Thus, as we attempt to locate or recognize one of these medications using the picture we have developed in our mind, we may be unable to see any disconfirming evidence if the wrong product is selected. Instead, we see the drug we intend to see.

For example, glance at the image below. What do you see?

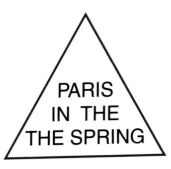

Many people see PARIS IN THE SPRING. However, the word THE appears twice, and can easily be overlooked if people are familiar with the phrase and expect to see it written just as they envision it in their mind.

Now look at the following image. What do you see?

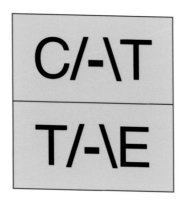

Most likely, you read the top word as CAT and the bottom word as THE, even though the middle character making up the A in CAT and the H in THE is identical and cannot logically represent both letters. Words, including drug names, are initially perceived as a whole, with comprehension occurring first at the word level and then moving down to the individual letters. Thus, a drug name will be read in its entirety first; then individual letters might be randomly sampled to confirm your expectations. However, if you expect to see the name of a specific medication, you will likely confirm that expectation even if some of the letters are wrong.

Examples of Look-Alike/Sound-Alike Medications [16A]

Listed below are examples of drug name pairs that have been involved in errors related to similar pronunciation or appearance.

DRUG	CONFUSED WITH
ABELCET	amphotericin B
ACTIVASE	TNKase
ADDERALL	INDERAL
amphotericin B	AMBISOME
aripiprazole	Drugs in the class of Proton Pump Inhibitors
aripiprazole	rabeprazole
COMVAX	RECOMBIVAX HB
daptomycin	dactinomycin
DEPAKOTE ER	DEPAKOTE
DEPO-MEDROL	SOLU-MEDROL
DIPRIVAN	DITROPAN
dobutamine	dopamine
ENDOCET	INDOCID
ephedrine	epinephrine
EPO (epoetin alfa)	EPO (evening primrose oil)
folinic acid (leucovorin calcium)	folic acid
heparin	HESPAN
HUMALOG	HUMULIN
HYDROGESIC	hydroxyzine
"K" (potassium)	vitamin K
KALETRA	KEPPRA
LANOXIN	levothyroxine
LANTUS	LENTE
leucovorin calcium	LEUKERAN
LEXAPRO	LOXITANE
LIPITOR	ZYRTEC
MgSO4 (magnesium sulfate)	MSO4 (morphine)
METADATE	methadone
METADATE ER	METADATE CD
NARCAN	NORCURON
propylthiouracil	PURINETHOL
RITALIN LA	RITALIN SR
SEROQUEL	SERZONE

continued

Examples of Look-Alike/Sound-Alike Medications (continued)

sertraline	SORIATANE
SSRI (sliding scale regular insulin)	SSRI (selective serotonin reuptake inhibitor)
TAXOL	TAXOTERE
tizanidine	tiagabine
TNKase	t-PA
TRACLEER	TRICOR
trazodone	tramadol
TYLENOL PM	TYLENOL
VARIVAX	VZIG
WELLBUTRIN SR	WELLBUTRIN XL
ZEBETA	ZETIA
ZESTRIL	ZETIA
ZOSTRIX	ZOVIRAX
ZYPREXA	ZYRTEC

Uppercase, brand name; **lowercase**, generic name.

■ SAFETY STRATEGIES ■

Tall Man Lettering

One way to encourage healthcare providers to focus on the individual letters that distinguish one drug name from another is to use **tall man lettering**. This technique enhances the unique letter characters of look-alike drug names by using upper case letters. The Food and Drug Administration (Office of Generic Drugs) has requested that manufacturers of sixteen look-alike generic drug name pairs voluntarily revise their appearance, using tall man letters, in order to minimize medication errors resulting from look-alike confusion.

FDA List of Generic Look-Alike Names and Recommended Revisions[2]

LOOK-ALIKE DRUG NAME PAIRS	SUGGESTED USE OF TALL MAN LETTERS
acetazolamide	aceta**ZOLAMIDE**
acetohexamide	aceto**HEXAMIDE**
bupropion	bu**PROP**ion
buspirone	bus**PIR**one
chlorpromazine	chlorpro**MAZINE**
chlorpropamide	chlorpro**PAMIDE**
clomiphene	clomi**PHENE**
clomipramine	clomi**PRAMINE**
cyclosporine	cyclo**SPORINE**
cycloserine	cyclo**SERINE**
daunorubicin	**DAUNO**rubicin
doxorubicin	**DOXO**rubicin
dimenhydrinate	dimenhy**DRINATE**
diphenhydramine	diphenhydr**AMINE**
dobutamine	**DOBUT**amine
dopamine	**DOP**amine
glipizide	glipi**ZIDE**
glyburide	gly**BURIDE**
hydralazine	hydr**ALAZINE**
hydroxyzine	hydr**OXY**zine
medroxyprogesterone	medroxy**PROGESTER**one
methylprednisolone	methyl**PREDNIS**olone
methyltestosterone	methyl**TESTOSTER**one
nicardipine	ni**CAR**dipine
nifedipine	**NIFE**dipine
prednisone	predni**SONE**
prednisolone	predniso**LONE**
sulfadiazine	sulf**ADIAZINE**
sulfisoxazole	sulfi**SOXAZOLE**
tolazamide	**TOLAZ**amide
tolbutamide	**TOLBUT**amide
vinblastine	vin**BLAS**tine
vincristine	vin**CRIS**tine

Safety Strategies for Look-/Sound-Alike Drug Names or Look-Alike Packages[22,24A]

SAFETY PROBLEM	SAFETY STRATEGIES
	Look-Alike Names (Brand or Generic)
Differentiate items	• For name pairs known to be problematic, include both generic and brand names on orders, storage shelves and product labels, computer screens, and MARs • Change the appearance of look-alike names on storage shelves and product labels, computer screens, and MARs by using color, bold face, and/or tall man lettering (e.g., hydrOXYzine, hydrALAzine) • When feasible, use magnifying lenses and good lighting during transcription to improve the likelihood of proper interpretation of look-alike product names • Do not list medications with look-alike names sequentially on computer screens, preprinted order forms, or MARs
Improve access to information	• Include the drug's indication on all prn orders • Match the purpose of the medication to the patient's specific diagnoses before administering it (many products with look-alike names are used for different purposes)
Use reminders	• Affix "name alert" stickers to areas where look-alike products are stored
Redundancies	• Require pharmacy to review all medication orders before drug administration whenever possible • Engage the patient in a double check; make sure the medication's intended purpose makes sense to the patient and that the medication looks similar to prior doses administered or taken at home • Investigate if the patient suggests the medication does not look similar in appearance to prior doses

Simplify	• Accept verbal/telephone orders only when truly necessary
Standardize	• Prohibit all verbal/telephone orders for selected high-alert medications such as antineoplastics
	• Require staff who accept verbal/telephone orders to write them immediately as received onto the patient's chart
Redundancies	• Read back all transcribed verbal/oral orders, spelling drug names, stating numerical doses in single digits (one-five, not fifteen), and stating the drug's intended purpose to verify understanding
Use reminders	• Affix "name alert" stickers to areas where sound-alike products are stored
Look-Alike Packaging	
Differentiate items	• Purchase products with look-alike packaging from different manufacturers
	• Circle important information on the package to draw attention to differences
Limit access or use	• Segregate medications with look-alike packages by storing in separate areas
	• Return medications to their segregated storage area after use (e.g., multiple-use vials of insulin, heparin)
Use reminders	• Add shelf stickers to draw attention to the medication's name
	• Add look-alike alert stickers to problematic medications in look-alike packaging
	• Build look-alike alerts to appear on the screen of automated dispensing cabinets for problematic medications in look-alike packages

continued

Safety Strategies for Look-/Sound-Alike Drug Names or Look-Alike Packages (continued)

SAFETY PROBLEM	SAFETY STRATEGIES
	Look-Alike Packaging
Redundancies	• Require pharmacy to review all medication orders before drug administration whenever possible • Engage the patient in a double check; make sure the medication's intended purpose makes sense to the patient and that the medication looks similar to prior doses administered or taken at home • Investigate if the patient suggests the medication does not look similar in appearance to prior doses
	New Medications
Failure mode and effects analysis (FMEA)*	• Anticipate the possibility of errors with new medications due to a name that looks or sounds like another product already in use or a package that looks similar to another medication already in use • Perform a FMEA for new high-alert medications before use

*Additional information on FMEA can be found in **Assessing Risk**.

Key terms highlighted in **green** throughout
the text are defined in the **Glossary**.

Error-Prone Abbreviations, Symbols, and Dose Expressions[20]

Abbreviations and symbols may appear to be a great time saver but their use can be problematic when used to communicate medical information.

- An abbreviation or symbol may have more than one meaning.
- The reader may be unfamiliar with the intended meaning of the abbreviation or symbol.
- If poorly written, an abbreviation or symbol may be mistaken for another abbreviation or symbol.
- There is considerable variation in the abbreviations and symbols used for common medical terms.

Error-prone methods of expressing doses have also contributed to serious dosing errors. For example, ten-fold overdoses have resulted from the failure to include a zero before the decimal point for doses less than a whole unit (.1 instead of 0.1), or the addition of an unnecessary decimal point and zero for whole number doses (1.0 instead of 1).

Examples in Practice[44-48]

The following are examples of errors introduced by abbreviations. In the first case, the order was interpreted as 25 "u" (units) per hour, but that wasn't the physician's intent. He wrote *25 cc/hour*, intending a 1,000 unit/hour dose using the hospital's standard heparin concentration of 20,000 units/500 mL (40 units/mL). Certainly, prescribing the dose in units would have been safer. Fortunately, the rate in mL/hour was so low that the mistake was quickly recognized. If only 25 units/hour had been given, the patient would have received a mere 2.5% of the prescribed dose.

$$25 \, u/h$$

An order was written on a weekend for a 70-year-old leukemic patient to receive "vincristine .4 mg qd x 4 d". A 4 mg vincristine dose was prepared and given to the patient. Even though the patient received a ten-fold overdose for one day of therapy, the patient suffered no permanent injury.

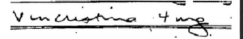

The prescriber intended the patient to receive Lovenox 40 mg daily. However, his use of the error-prone abbreviation "QD" for daily led a nurse to misinterpret this order as Lovenox 40 mg "Q8" hours, even though the medication is typically administered daily or every 12 hours.

"QD" also is frequently misinterpreted as "QID" (four times daily), as demonstrated in the next order. The raised tail on the q led to misreading "qd" as "qid."

In this case, an order for an infusion with sodium bicarbonate to run "@50 cc/h" was misread as 250 mL per hour.

A patient with renal failure was given a dose of vancomycin along with orders to administer another 1 g dose intravenously if his vancomycin level was "less than 10" the next morning. The following day, a nurse called the pharmacy to ask if a level of "35" was close enough to give the next dose. The nurse was told to hold the vancomycin until the pharmacist could investigate why she thought a serum level of 35 mcg/mL was "close enough" to 10 mcg/mL. A quick look at the original order revealed the nurse's source of confusion. The symbol for "less than" was written in a way that made the number 10 look more like 40. A more acceptable way to write such an order is, "If morning vancomycin level is less than 10 mcg/mL, give a single 1 g dose of vancomycin IVPB."

if Am Vancomycin level is <10, give 1 nm IV. 1 dose

Historically, to address these issues, many healthcare providers have maintained a list of approved abbreviations, symbols, and dose expressions for use within an organization. A much more efficient alternative is to maintain a list of error-prone abbreviations, symbols, and dose expressions that should NEVER be used.

The following tables contain error-prone abbreviations, symbols, and dose designations that have been involved in harmful medication errors. They should NEVER be used in handwritten, preprinted, or electronic forms of communication, including orders, MAR entries, preprinted orders, labels, and computer screens.

Joint Commission Requirements[29]

One of the 2004 Joint Commission National Patient Safety Goals requires compliance with prohibiting all the abbreviations and dose designations specified with a double asterisk (**) in the following tables, along with at least three other items from the lists. However, we hope that you will consider others beyond the minimum Joint Commission requirement.

Error-Prone Abbreviations[13]

ABBREVIATIONS	INTENDED MEANING	MISINTERPRETATION	CORRECTION
μg	Microgram	Mistaken as "mg"	Use "mcg"
AD, AS, AU	Right ear, left ear, each ear	Mistaken as "OD", "OS", "OU" (right eye, left eye, each eye)	Use "right ear," "left ear," or "each ear"
OD, OS, OU	Right eye, left eye, each eye	Mistaken as "AD", "AS", "AU" (right ear, left ear, each ear)	Use "right eye," "left eye," or "each eye"
BT	Bedtime	Mistaken as "BID" (twice daily)	Use "bedtime"
cc	Cubic centimeters	Mistaken as "u" (units)	Use "mL"
D/C	Discharge or discontinue	Premature discontinuation of medications if D/C (intended to mean "discharge") has been misinterpreted as "discontinued" when followed by a list of discharge medications	Use "discharge" and "discontinue"
IJ	Injection	Mistaken as "IV" or "intrajugular"	Use "injection"
IN	Intranasal	Mistaken as "IM" or "IV"	Use "intranasal" or "NAS"
HS	Half-strength	Mistaken as "bedtime"	Use "half-strength" or "bedtime"
hs	At bedtime, hours of sleep	Mistaken as "half-strength"	Use "half-strength" or "bedtime"
IU**	International unit	Mistaken as "IV" (intravenous) or "10" (ten)	Use "units"

continued

Error-Prone Abbreviations (continued)

ABBREVIATIONS	INTENDED MEANING	MISINTERPRETATION	CORRECTION
o.d. or OD	Once daily	Mistaken as "right eye" (OD, oculus dexter), leading to oral liquid medications administered in the eye	Use "daily"
OJ	Orange juice	Mistaken as "OD" or "OS" (right or left eye); drugs meant to be diluted in orange juice may be given in the eye	Use "orange juice"
Per os	By mouth, orally	The "os" can be mistaken as "left eye" (OS, oculus sinister)	Use "PO," "by mouth," or "orally"
q.d. or QD**	Every day	Mistaken as "q.i.d.", especially if period after the "q" or tail of the "q" is misunderstood as an "i"	Use "daily"
qhs	At bedtime	Mistaken as "qhr" (every hour)	Use "at bedtime"
qn	Nightly	Mistaken as "qh" (every hour)	Use "nightly"
q.o.d. or QOD**	Every other day	Mistaken as "q.d." (daily) or "q.i.d." (four times daily) if the "o" is poorly written	Use "every other day"
q1d	Daily	Mistaken as "q.i.d." (four times daily)	Use "daily"
q6PM, etc.	Every evening at 6 PM	Mistaken as every 6 hours	Use "6 PM nightly" or "6 PM daily"

64

SC, SQ, sub q	Subcutaneous	SC mistaken as "SL" (sublingual); SQ mistaken as "5 every"; the "q" in "sub q" has been mistaken as "every" (e.g., a heparin dose ordered "sub q 2 hours before surgery" misunderstood as every 2 hours before surgery)	Use "subcut" or "subcutaneously"
ss	Sliding scale (insulin) or ½ (apothecary)	Mistaken as "55"	Spell out "sliding scale" Use "one-half" or "½"
SSRI	Sliding scale regular insulin	Mistaken as selective serotonin reuptake inhibitor	Spell out "sliding scale (insulin)"
SSI	Sliding scale insulin	Mistaken as Strong Solution of Iodine (Lugol's)	Spell out "sliding scale (insulin)"
1/d	One daily	Mistaken as "tid"	Use "1 daily"
TIW or tiw	3 times a week	Mistaken as "3 times a day" or "twice in a week"	Use "3 times weekly"
U or u**	Unit	Mistaken as the number 0 or 4, causing a 10-fold overdose or greater (e.g., 4U seen as "40" or 4u seen as "44"); mistaken as "cc" so dose given in volume instead of units (e.g., 4u seen as 4cc)	Use "unit"

**Identified abbreviations above are also included on Joint Commission's "minimum list" of dangerous abbreviations, acronyms, and symbols that must be included on an organization's "Do Not Use" list, effective January 1, 2004. An updated list of frequently asked questions about this Joint Commission requirement can be found on their website at www.jcaho.org.

Error-Prone Dose Designations [13]

DOSE DESIGNATIONS AND OTHER INFORMATION	INTENDED MEANING	MISINTERPRETATION	CORRECTION
Trailing zero after decimal point (e.g., 1.0 mg)**	1 mg	Mistaken as 10 mg if the decimal point is not seen	Do not use trailing zeros for doses expressed in whole numbers
No leading zero before a decimal dose (e.g., .5 mg)	0.5 mg	Mistaken as 5 mg if the decimal point is not seen	Use zero before a decimal point when the dose is less than a whole unit
Drug name and dose run together (e.g., drug names ending in "L"—Inderal40 mg; Tegretol300 mg)	Inderal 40 mg Tegretol 300 mg	Mistaken as Inderal 140 mg Mistaken as Tegretol 1300 mg	Place adequate space between the drug name, dose, and unit of measure
Numerical dose and unit of measure run together (e.g., 10mg, 100mL)	10 mg 100 mL	The "m" is sometimes mistaken as a zero or two zeros, risking a 10- to 100-fold overdose	Place adequate space between the dose and unit of measure
Period following an abbreviation (e.g., mg. or mL.)	mg mL	The period is unnecessary and could be mistaken as the number 1	Use mg, mL, etc. without a terminal period

| Large doses without properly placed commas (e.g., **100000** units; **1000000 units**) | 100,000 units 1,000,000 units | 100000 has been mistaken as 10,000 or 1,000,000; 1000000 has been mistaken as 100,000 | Use commas for dosing units at or above 1,000, or use words such as 100 "thousand" or 1 "million" to improve |

**Identified dose designations above are also included on Joint Commission's "minimum list" of dangerous abbreviations, acronyms, and symbols that must be included on an organization's "Do Not Use" list, effective January 1, 2004. An updated list of frequently asked questions about this Joint Commission requirement can be found on their website at www.jcaho.org.

Error-Prone Drug Stems[13]			
STEMMED DRUG NAMES	**INTENDED MEANING**	**MISINTERPRETATION**	**CORRECTION**
"Nitro" drip	nitroglycerin infusion	Mistaken as sodium nitroprusside infusion	Use complete drug name
"Norflox"	norfloxacin	Mistaken as Norflex	Use complete drug name
"IV Vanc"	intravenous vancomycin	Mistaken as Invanz	Use complete drug name

Error-Prone Drug Name Abbreviations [13]

DRUG NAME ABBREVIATIONS	INTENDED MEANING	MISINTERPRETATION	CORRECTION
ARA A	vidarabine	Mistaken as cytarabine (ARA C)	Use complete drug name
AZT	zidovudine (Retrovir)	Mistaken as azathioprine or aztreonam	Use complete drug name
CPZ	Compazine (prochlorperazine)	Mistaken as chlorpromazine	Use complete drug name
DPT	Demerol-Phenergan-Thorazine	Mistaken as diphtheria-pertussis-tetanus (vaccine)	Use complete drug name
DTO	Diluted tincture of opium, or deodorized tincture of opium (Paregoric)	Mistaken as tincture of opium	Use complete drug name
HCl	hydrochloric acid or hydrochloride	Mistaken as potassium chloride ("H" is misinterpreted as "K")	Use complete drug name unless expressed as salt of a drug
HCT	hydrocortisone	Mistaken as hydrochlorothiazide	Use complete drug name
HCTZ	hydrochlorothiazide	Mistaken as hydrocortisone (seen as HCT250 mg)	Use complete drug name
MgSO4**	magnesium sulfate	Mistaken as morphine sulfate	Use complete drug name
MS, MSO4**	morphine sulfate	Mistaken as magnesium sulfate	Use complete drug name

68

MTX	methotrexate	Mistaken as mitoxantrone	Use complete drug name
PCA	procainamide	Mistaken as Patient Controlled Analgesia	Use complete drug name
PTU	propylthiouracil	Mistaken as mercaptopurine	Use complete drug name
T3	Tylenol with codeine No. 3	Mistaken as liothyronine	Use complete drug name
TAC	triamcinolone	Mistaken as tetracaine, Adrenalin, cocaine	Use complete drug name
TNK	TNKase	Mistaken as "TPA"	Use complete drug name
ZnSO4	zinc sulfate	Mistaken as morphine sulfate	Use complete drug name

**Identified drug name abbreviations above are also included on Joint Commission's "minimum list" of dangerous abbreviations, acronyms, and symbols that must be included on an organization's "Do Not Use" list, effective January 1, 2004. An updated list of frequently asked questions about this Joint Commission requirement can be found on their website at www.jcaho.org.

Error-Prone Symbols[13]

SYMBOLS	INTENDED MEANING	MISINTERPRETATION	CORRECTION
℥	Dram	Symbol for dram mistaken as "3"	Use the metric system
♏	Minim	Symbol for minim mistaken as "mL"	Use the metric system
x3d	For three days	Mistaken as "3 doses"	Use "for three days"
> and <	Greater than and less than	Mistaken as opposite of intended; mistakenly use incorrect symbol; "<10" mistaken as "40"	Use "greater than" or "less than"
/ (slash mark)	Separates two doses or indicates "per"	Mistaken as "1" (e.g., "25 units/10 units" misread as "25 units and 110" units)	Use "per" rather than a slash mark to separate doses
@	At	Mistaken as "2"	Use "at"
&	And	Mistaken as "2"	Use "and"
+	Plus or and	Mistaken as "4"	Use "and"
°	Hour	Mistaken as a zero (e.g., q2° seen as q20)	Use "hr," "h," or "hour"

HIGH-RISK PROCESSES

SEE ALSO

High-Risk

Key terms highlighted in **green** throughout
the text are defined in the **Glossary**.

CHARACTERISTICS[28]

A high-risk process, much like a high-risk medication, is one in which a failure of some kind is most likely to jeopardize the safety of the patient or the staff member involved.

Typically, high-risk processes have several, if not all, of the following characteristics:

- **Complexity** – the process consists of a lot of steps and handoffs between multiple people
- **Non-standard** – the process is often performed differently by various people with mixed levels of success
- **Rigid sequencing** – the process must be carried out in a specific sequence; each step is dependent on achievement of the prior step, and thus a change in order will result in failure
- **Time sensitivity** – the process cannot tolerate delays within each step of the process or in completion of the process
- **Variable recipients** – the process is carried out for many different patients who have a mix of disease states, varying in severity
- **Variable workers** – the process is carried out by workers who have differing levels of experience and knowledge
- **Cascading failures** – a small mistake in one step of the process clearly affects the rest of the process, often causing large failures in the end

High-risk processes are more likely to fail when carried out in an environment where intimidation, hierarchical roles, and fear of failure hinder effective communication, collaboration, and teamwork.

EXAMPLES IN MEDICATION USE

- Communication of orders to pharmacy

- Delivery of medications to patient units

- Order entry/transcription process

- Epidural or intrathecal drug administration

- Mixing IV solutions

- Programming infusion pumps

- Accurate bar code on all medications

- Mathematical calculations

- Dosing for pediatric patients

- Use of drug samples

Detailed strategies for managing these high-risk processes follow:

- Verbal/telephone orders

- Use of automated dispensing equipment

- Patient-controlled analgesia

Safety Strategies for Accepting and Transcribing Verbal/Telephone Orders[12A]

Safety Problem: Overuse of verbal orders

Causative Factors: convenience, habit, poor access to patient record, insufficient environment and space

SAFETY STRATEGIES	EXAMPLES
Limit use	• Reserve verbal orders for true emergencies or when the prescriber is physically unable to write or electronically transmit orders (e.g., working in a sterile field) • Prohibit all verbal/telephone orders for selected high-alert medications (e.g., antineoplastics, IV insulin for neonates) • In a hospital setting, limit verbal orders to medications on the drug formulary
Simplify	• Establish standing orders with corresponding preprinted order forms for areas where verbal/telephone orders tend to be prevalent (e.g., ED, critical care units) • Provide physician offices with appropriate order forms and request transmission of orders for new admissions via fax, pneumatic tube, or electronically, rather than by telephone
Improve access	• Locate and hand the patient's medical record to any prescriber who is attempting to issue verbal orders while physically present in the unit (and capable of writing/entering the orders) • Stock order forms in patient records for easy access • Provide adequate space (and computer terminals, as appropriate) for prescribers in a low-traffic area

Safety Problem: Mistranscribed telephone/verbal orders	
Causative Factors: delayed transcription, chart unavailability, mental slip, transcribed onto the wrong patient's chart	
SAFETY STRATEGIES	EXAMPLES
Simplify	• Document a verbal/telephone order directly onto the patient's medical record immediately, while it is being received, before reading the order back for verification
Redundancies	• To verify patient identity, read back the patient's name on the order form that was used to transcribe the verbal/telephone order
	• If taking a telephone order, obtain the prescriber's phone number for questions that arise

Safety Problem: Misheard, misinterpreted, or fraudulent verbal/telephone orders	
Causative Factors: sound-alike drug names, sound-alike numbers, momentary inattention, distractions, noise, phone interference, hearing impairment, unfamiliarity with prescriber and prescriber's voice	
SAFETY STRATEGIES	EXAMPLES
Limit Use (Access)	• Limit the number of nurses who may receive telephone orders to maximize the ability to recognize the caller's voice (which reduces the risk of fraudulent telephone orders)

continued

Safety Strategies for Accepting and Transcribing Verbal/Telephone Orders (continued)

Redundancies	• After writing the order on the patient record (immediately as received), read back the entire order as documented to the prescriber for confirmation
	• Spell all drug names
	• Confirm numbers using single digits ("one-four" for 14, "one-zero" for 10)
	• Ask for the drug's indication, or communicate your understanding of its intended purpose to further ensure accuracy
	• Make sure the medication makes sense in context of the patient's condition
	• If the medication prescribed requires emergency administration (or the nurse is working within a sterile field), repeat back the order as above, and also announce the medication again just before administration ("I am now giving heparin 2,000 units IV") if the prescriber is at the patient's bedside

Safety Strategies for Patient Controlled Analgesia [18,19A]

Safety Problem: PCA by proxy – when someone other than the patient presses the button to deliver a dose of medication
Causative Factors: desire to keep patients comfortable without knowledge that PCA by proxy could lead to oversedation, respiratory arrest, or death

SAFETY STRATEGIES	EXAMPLES
Improve access to information	• Educate patients about the proper use of PCA; start during the preoperative testing visit so patients are not too groggy to understand
Limit access	• Warn caregivers, family members, and visitors about the dangers of PCA by proxy • Identify the infrequent situations in which critical care patients may be suitable for nurse-controlled analgesia (nurse delivers each dose), and the level of enhanced monitoring required for these patients
Use reminders	• Place warning labels on activation buttons that state "FOR PATIENT USE ONLY" • Provide visual and auditory feedback to patients when the button is pressed

Safety Problem: Improper patient selection – allowing patients who do not have the mental alertness, cognitive ability, or physical capacity to safely manage their own pain
Causative Factors: desire to quickly administer pain medication, leading to PCA by proxy (see above)

SAFETY STRATEGIES	EXAMPLES
Limit use	• Establish patient selection criteria; candidates should have an appropriate level of consciousness and cognitive ability to manage their pain; infants, young children, and confused or agitated patients are not suitable candidates

continued

Safety Strategies for Patient Controlled Analgesia (continued)

Safety Problem: Inadequate patient monitoring – typical monitoring activities may not alert caregivers to opioid toxicity

Causative Factors: failure to notice depth/quality of respirations when taking vital signs; overreliance on routine vital signs, observation after physical stimulus, and pulse oximetry to detect adverse effects of the drug (e.g., oversedation, depressed respirations, heart rate, blood pressure)

SAFETY STRATEGIES	EXAMPLES
Patient monitoring	• At minimum, evaluate pain, alertness, and vital signs (include respiratory quality and depth) every 4 hours • Monitor patients more frequently during the first 24 hours and at night (when hypoventilation and nocturnal hypoxia can occur) • Evaluate patients with minimal verbal and tactile stimulation to obtain an accurate assessment of their level of sedation • Establish risk factors that could increase respiratory depression (e.g., obesity, low body weight, concomitant medications that potentiate opioids, asthma, sleep apnea) and determine the level of enhanced monitoring required (e.g., capnography, apnea alarms at night) • Require special monitoring (e.g., more frequent observation, vital signs, capnography) in the rare instances that nurse-controlled PCA is employed • Do not rely on pulse oximetry readings alone to detect opioid toxicity (oxygen saturation is usually maintained even at low respiratory rates)

| | • Keep PCA flowsheets at the bedside to document PCA doses and patient monitoring |
| | • Have oxygen and naloxone readily available at the bedside in the event of oversedation or respiratory depression |

Safety Problem: Drug product mix-ups – selecting the wrong concentration or the wrong drug when preparing PCA (e.g., morphine is available in both a 1 mg/mL and a 5 mg/mL concentration; morphine and hydromorphone have been confused)

Causative Factors: similar drug names, packages, and labels; ambiguous drug labels

SAFETY STRATEGIES	EXAMPLES
Standardize	• Establish one standard concentration for each opioid used for PCA
	• Use prefilled syringes/bags/cassettes whenever available commercially; have pharmacy mix all PCA products that are not commercially available (hydromorphone)
Limit access	• Stock only the standard concentrations for morphine and hydromorphone in patient care units (dispense any other drugs used for PCA from the pharmacy)
	• Separate the storage of morphine and hydromorphone to avoid mix-ups
Use reminders	• Ask pharmacy to affix prominent warnings if dispensing an opioid in a nonstandard concentration
Differentiate items	• Ask pharmacy to use tall man lettering for HYDROmorphone to differentiate it from morphine
Require redundancies	• Require pharmacy to review all PCA orders before initiation
	• Require an independent double check for patient identification, drug and concentration, pump settings, and the line attachment before initiation of PCA, and at each syringe/cassette/dose change
	• Employ bar coding to verify the drug and concentration

continued

Safety Strategies for Patient Controlled Analgesia (continued)

Safety Problem: Prescribing errors – prescribing the wrong drug or dose, or prescribing an opioid to which the patient is allergic

Causative Factors: mistakes during dose conversion (oral to IV), especially for hydromorphone; other calculation errors; lack of information about patient allergies; unrecognized prescriptions for other opioids

SAFETY STRATEGIES	EXAMPLES
Standardize and simplify	• Accept PCA orders only from prescribers who possess requisite proficiency • Use standard order sets to guide drug selection, doses, and lockout periods; patient monitoring; and precautions such as avoiding concomitant analgesics (which should also appear on the MAR) • Accept verbal/telephone orders only for dose changes • Ensure that prescribers have a list of other medications that the patient has received (e.g., at home, intraoperatively) for consideration when determining the loading dose • Use morphine as opioid of choice; use hydromorphone for patients needing very high doses

Safety Problem: PCA device misprogramming

Causative Factors: lack of training, unfamiliarity with various pumps, error-prone programming process, failure to include frontline nurses (pump users) in decisions regarding the purchase of pumps

SAFETY STRATEGIES	EXAMPLES
Improve access to information	• Train nurses to program PCA pumps and offer practice sessions as needed to maintain proficiency • Provide laminated instructions for use that are attached to each pump
Limit access (reduce options)	• Limit PCA pumps to a single model to promote proficiency
Forcing functions and fail-safes	• Establish default settings on the PCA pump of zero or the highest concentration available for opioids used to deliver PCA
Require redundancies	• Require an independent double check for patient identification, drug and concentration, pump settings, and the line attachment before initiation of PCA, and at each syringe/cassette/dose change • Verify PCA settings each shift, immediately after receiving report • Use "smart" PCA pumps that will immediately alert the nurse if a programming error has been made
Failure mode and effects analysis	• Include frontline nurses in the evaluation of new PCA pumps under consideration for purchase to help identify potential failure points (see **Assessing Risk** for sample questions to guide this process)

81

Safety Strategies for Automated Dispensing Cabinets [15,17,21A]

Safety Problem: Removing and administering non-urgent medications before a pharmacist has reviewed the order
Causative Factor: cabinets not linked to the pharmacy, need for urgent or emergency administration of medications, unacceptable delay in pharmacy processing of orders, workflow convenience

SAFETY STRATEGIES	EXAMPLES
Limit access	• Ensure that cabinets are linked electronically to the pharmacy, so pharmacists can enter and screen orders before drugs (especially high-alert medications) are removed and administered • Establish a restricted list of drugs that may be obtained via an override feature • Before nurses access a medication available via an override feature, require them to ask: Does the clinical need for quick administration outweigh the safety of the pharmacist reviewing the order first? • Require nurses to be "certified" via special education before accessing a medication via an override feature • Stock drugs available via an override feature separately from those that require pharmacy review before access
Require redundancies	• Routinely review the list of drugs obtained via an override feature to determine that an appropriate reason existed • Require an independent check (two nurses) to confirm any high-alert medication removed from the cabinet via an override feature

82

Improve access to information	• Ensure timely delivery of all orders to the pharmacy for processing • Ensure timely order verification by pharmacy to prevent treatment delays

Safety Problem: Selecting the wrong medication, the wrong dose/concentration/form, or a duplicate dose

(a drug that has been removed and administered to the patient already)

Causative Factors: knowledge deficit about the drug; insufficient information about the patient (e.g., weight, allergies, age, renal status); look-alike names, packages, and labels on drug products; ambiguous labels on drugs; cabinet stocking error; delayed documentation of drug administration

SAFETY STRATEGIES	EXAMPLES
Limit access	• Carefully select medications stocked in the cabinets on the basis of the needs of each unit and the age and diagnoses of the patients being treated • Stock medications in limited quantities, single concentrations, and in ready-to-use, unit-dose packages • Place high-alert drugs in individual bins (no other drugs available in drawer) • Separate pediatric and adult concentrations of medications stocked in cabinets (preferably a separate cabinet for each)
Improve access to information	• Read medication labels aloud, holding the item first in one hand, then after switching the item to the other hand (to improve ability to read labels correctly without confirmation bias — see **Look-Alike Drugs** for more information)

continued

Safety Strategies for Automated Dispensing Cabinets (continued)

Use reminders	• Program important alerts so they appear on access screens (e.g., allergy alert, dose alert, route alert) especially for high-alert medications and drugs available via an override feature • Establish an alert on the access screen if an attempt is made to remove a medication that has recently been removed for the same patient • Affix auxiliary warnings to products to remind nurses about special precautions that could be life threatening if not carried out
Use forcing functions	• Require allergy verification before removal of medications such as opioids, antibiotics, and NSAIDs
Require redundancies	• Require an independent check (two nurses) to confirm selected high-alert medications removed from the cabinet • Require a check system for pharmacy restocking of the cabinets • Employ bar coding technology when stocking and selecting medications from the cabinet to ensure accuracy
Standardize and simplify	• Allow only trained pharmacy staff to replenish cabinets • Allow nurses to remove only a single dose of the medication ordered • Prohibit nurses from restocking unused drugs to original bin; provide a restock bin

NSAIDs, nonsteroidal anti-inflammatory drugs.

SEE ALSO

➤ **DO NOT USE**

➤ **HIGH-RISK PROCESSES**

Assessing
Risk

Key terms highlighted in **green** throughout
the text are defined in the **Glossary**.

■ PROACTIVE RISK ASSESSMENT ■

Use of the Ten Key Elements to Assess Risk

Frontline nurses play an essential role in assessing risk in their organizations because they, more than any other clinician, have firsthand experience with many of the error-prone systems and processes that affect their patients. Medication administration is no exception.

To help uncover the hidden risks often associated with medication administration, ask yourself the following questions every day when administering medications. This will aid you in identifying risks so that action can be taken to prevent errors and the patient harm that can result.

Assessing Risk – An Evaluation Tool for Frontline Nurses [1A]

SYSTEM ELEMENT	QUESTIONS TO CONSIDER
Patient information (e.g., patient identity, age, gender, diagnoses, pregnancy, allergies, height, weight, lab values, diagnostic study results, vital signs, ability to pay for prescriptions) *Essential patient information is obtained, readily available in useful form, and considered when prescribing, dispensing, and administering medications.*	• Does our information technology system provide easy electronic access to all patient laboratory information at any terminal with password entry? • Do all patients have bar-coded name bracelets and color-coded allergy bracelets? • Are allergies clearly visible on all order forms, MARs, and patient charts? • Have I provided the pharmacy with the patient's allergies, recent weight (and any weight changes), and pregnancy status? • Will the pharmacist be able to read the patient's name and other important demographic information on the order after it is transmitted to the pharmacy? • Do I always take the patient's MAR to the bedside for a final verification of the patient's identity, allergies, and drug therapy?
Drug information (e.g. maximum dose, typical dose, route, precautions, contraindications, special warnings, drug interactions, cross allergies)	• Do I have *only* the most current drug references on my unit (no outdated texts)? • Do I have easy access to online drug information resources on all terminals on my unit? • Are special precautions such as dosing charts, auxiliary labels, and protocols with mixing instructions available to me for high-alert medications? • Are pharmacists physically present and readily available on my unit to assist with medication choices, answer questions, and participate in patient education?

continued

Assessing Risk - An Evaluation Tool for Frontline Nurses *(continued)*

SYSTEM ELEMENT	QUESTIONS TO CONSIDER
Essential drug information is readily available in a useful form when ordering, dispensing, or administering medications.	• Are all preprinted order sets and protocols current and updated at least annually? • Does a pharmacist screen all medication orders, where possible, before medications are available to me for administration?
Communication (e.g., communication dynamics among colleagues, team dynamics, communication of drug orders) *Methods of communicating drug orders and other drug information are standardized and automated to minimize the risk for error.*	• Do I immediately write down all verbal orders and repeat them back with spellings and single digits? • Do I refuse to accept verbal orders for antineoplastics? • Is the nursing MAR produced by pharmacy, and does it match the pharmacy profile? • Are medication administration times standardized on my unit? • Are there realistic timeframes established and followed for stat, now, and routine medication delivery? • Do I always call the prescriber when I have even vague concerns about the safety of an order? • Is there a hospital policy and procedure to resolve any conflicts if the prescriber disagrees with the expressed concerns about the safety of an order? • Do I avoid using error-prone abbreviations and dose expressions when transcribing medication orders? (See Tab **Do Not Use**)
Drug names, labels, and packages	• Do I label all syringes with the name and strength of the drug? • Do I label all drugs and solutions on the sterile field, even if only one product is in use?

Readable labels that clearly identify drugs and doses are on all medication containers, and drugs remain labeled up to the point of actual drug administration.	• Do I keep all oral medications in their original packaging until they reach the patient's bedside?
	• Are all medications dispensed to me in clearly labeled, unit-dose packages?
	• Do I understand all the information provided on the pharmacy-applied labels?
	• Are auxiliary warning labels placed on medications that contain odd strengths or doses?
Strategies are undertaken to minimize the possibility of errors with products that have similar or confusing labels/packages or drug names.	• Do I report any situations in which the package of one medication looks like the package of another medication?
	• Are medications with names that sound or look alike separated in storage areas, including automated dispensing cabinets?
Drug standardization, storage, and distribution (e.g., storage of unit stock medications and pharmacy-dispensed medications, preparation of IV medications, use of standard concentrations, pharmacy delivery services)	• Are only standard concentrations (preferably one) available for **high-alert medications**?
	• Are most IV solutions prepared by the manufacturer (premixed solutions)?
	• Does pharmacy prepare the majority of IV and oral medications (including oral solutions) in single, unit-dose packages that match the prescribed dose for the patient?
IV solutions, drug concentrations, and administration times are standardized whenever possible.	• Does pharmacy prepare all IV solutions that are not premixed from the manufacturer, except in true emergencies?
	• Does a process exist to remove discontinued medications in a timely manner?

continued

Assessing Risk - An Evaluation Tool for Frontline Nurses (continued)

SYSTEM ELEMENT	QUESTIONS TO CONSIDER
Medications are provided to patient care units in a safe and secure manner and available for administration within a time frame that meets essential patient needs. *Unit-based floor stock is restricted.*	• If high-alert medications are available on my unit, are they secured? • Is medication stock on my unit routinely reviewed by nursing and pharmacy? • Are nurses or other non-pharmacy staff prohibited from entering the pharmacy after hours if 24-hour service is not available? • Before removing a medication from an automated dispensing cabinet (or floor stock) via an override feature, do I always verify that the clinical need for quick administration outweighs the safety of having a pharmacist review the order first?
Medication delivery devices (e.g., infusion pumps, implantable pumps, oral and parenteral syringes, glucose monitors) *The potential for human error is mitigated through careful procurement, maintenance, use, and standardization of devices used to prepare and deliver medications.*	• Are all infusion pumps protected against accidental free-flow of solution if the tubing is removed from the pump? • Are nurses asked their opinion before new equipment and devices are used? • Do I review devices and supplies for error potential? • Are oral syringes that cannot be connected to IV tubing available and used on my unit? • Do I routinely label all infusion lines to prevent mix-ups? • Do I always get another practitioner to independently double check the IV solutions and pump settings for high-alert drugs?

Environmental factors and staffing patterns (e.g., physical surroundings, physical health of staff, organization of unit, lighting, noise, foot traffic, storage, ergonomics, workload, adequate staffing, safe work schedules) *Medications are prescribed, transcribed, prepared, and administered in a physical environment that offers adequate space and lighting, and allows practitioners to remain focused on medication use.* *The complement of qualified, well-rested practitioners matches the clinical workload without compromising patient safety.*	• Is there adequate space and lighting where I obtain stock medications (including at automated dispensing cabinets)? • Am I rarely interrupted when I am administering medications? • Is an area free of distractions available to me when I am transcribing medication orders and charting? • Am I prohibited from working longer than 12 hours, except in an emergency? • Do I rest for at least 10 hours between shifts? • Do I have the opportunity to take rest and meal breaks every shift? • Is staffing consistently adequate on my unit for the number and acuity of patients?
Staff competency and education (e.g., orientation, in-service training, certifications, annual competencies, skills labs, simulation of events, off-site education)	• Is medication safety part of orientation for all employees? • Am I provided with information on new medications prescribed for my patients? • If I am asked to precept new staff, are my patient duties curtailed? • Have I had an opportunity to learn pharmacy processes for medication preparation and dispensing?

continued

Assessing Risk · An Evaluation Tool for Frontline Nurses (continued)

SYSTEM ELEMENT	QUESTIONS TO CONSIDER
Practitioners receive sufficient orientation to medication use and undergo baseline and annual competency evaluation of knowledge and skills related to safe medication practices.	• Am I and other staff trained on how to respond to a medication error? • Does pharmacy or other education staff present in-services for new medications and medication error prevention?
Practitioners involved in medication use are provided with ongoing education about medication error prevention and the safe use of drugs that have the greatest potential to cause harm if misused.	
Patient education (e.g., drug information sheets, dosing schedules for complex medication regimens, discharge instructions, tips to avoid errors, consumer representation in drug safety efforts)	• Am I offered opportunities to attend off-site educational programs to maintain my skill level? • Do my patients know they play a part in safe medication use? • Do I encourage patients and caregivers to ask questions and to expect satisfaction from the answers provided? • Are my patients comfortable identifying themselves to hospital personnel and asking questions freely?

Patients are included as active partners in their care through education about their medications and ways to avert errors.	• Do I specifically instruct my patients to identify themselves before accepting medications?
	• Do I consider my patient's question carefully to determine if it could be a signal that something is wrong with the medication?
	• Do I always respond to questions with patience, accuracy, and in a timely fashion?
	• Do I hold off giving a medication until a satisfactory answer can be provided?
	• Do I always offer patients information about each medication during drug administration, especially for **high-alert medications**?
	• Do I avoid yes/no questions and ask patients to give me their own explanation of the material I have covered or to provide a repeat demonstration of skills?
	• Do I provide my patients with up-to-date, easy-to-read, printed materials about medications and medication safety?
	• Is my pharmacist available to teach patients about complex medication regimens or specific high-alert medications?
	• Do my patients know they can speak with a pharmacist?
Quality process and risk management (e.g., culture, leadership, error reporting, safety strategies, safety **redundancies**)	• Is the culture in the hospital blame-free concerning errors?
	• Do I freely report medication errors and near misses without fear of retribution?

continued

SYSTEM ELEMENT	QUESTIONS TO CONSIDER
A non-punitive, systems-based approach to error reduction is in place and supported by management, senior administration, and the Board of Trustees.	• Is there a person in my institution who has a leadership role for coordinating medication error prevention activities? • Do I disclose all medication errors that reach the patient? • Are incentives and positive feedback provided for individuals who report errors?
Practitioners are stimulated to detect and report errors, and interdisciplinary teams regularly analyze errors that have occurred within the organization and in other organizations for the purpose of redesigning systems to best support safe practitioner performance.	• Do administrators/senior managers regularly visit my unit and seek staff input on error prevention? • Do prescribers order pediatric medications in total dose and mg/kg dose, and antineoplastics in total dose and mg/m² or AUC dose? • Before administering a high-alert medication, do I ask another practitioner to perform an independent double check?
Simple redundancies that support a system of independent double checks or an automated verification process are used for vulnerable parts of the medication use process to detect and correct errors before they reach patients.	

Use of Failure Mode and Effects Analysis (FMEA) to Assess Risk in Processes

FMEA is a proactive process used to learn about risk, or potential failure points, in processes so that action can be taken to *prevent* errors, and especially to prevent patient harm. It begins with the assumption that anything that **can** go wrong **will** go wrong in carrying out critical processes.

Steps in a Failure Mode and Effects Analysis[28]

Identify a High-Risk Process to Analyze*

Assemble the FMEA team	• 6-8 persons with a diverse mix of knowledge about the different steps of the process • One person who is distanced from the process to provide fresh perspective
Diagram the process	• Using symbols and diagrams, describe the steps and decisions involved with carrying out this process • Show the interrelationships between other departments and staff members • Show the time sequence
Brainstorm potential failure modes and effects	**Part 1: Failure mode identification** • "What can go wrong with _____?" • Look at: people, materials, equipment, methods/procedures, information transfer, environment • Be creative **Part 2: Effects** • "For each failure mode, what are the potential effects on the patient or process?"
Prioritize the failure modes	• "How does it affect the patient, staff, facility?" (severity score: catastrophic, major, moderate, minor) • "What is the likelihood that it will happen?" (probability score: frequent, occasional, uncommon, remote)

Identify root causes of failure modes (at least failures that could cause harm to patients)	• Look for proximate causes – readily apparent, most immediate reasons for error, close to origin of failure mode, often related to human or equipment error • Look for root causes – systemic, far from origin of failure, existing across the organization
Redesign the process	**Goals:** • Prevent failure from happening • Prevent failure from reaching patient • Reduce harm if failure reaches patient **Methods:** • Creativity, leadership, willingness to change • Professional associations/expert guidelines • Literature review for how others have redesigned successfully
Analyze and test	• Start with simulations on paper, computer • Move to pilot testing on small scale: individual units, offices • Spread change to rest of organization
Implement and monitor	• Collect data using applicable indicators • Evaluate and modify the change(s) based on results

*See examples listed in **High-Risk Processes**.

Use of FMEA to Assess Risk with Medical Devices

While **FMEA** is often used to formally assess specific high-risk processes, the primary principles of FMEA can also be applied to the evaluation of medical devices. In fact, the healthcare FMEA process is derived from a much earlier FMEA process involved with the design of devices used in other industries. For this purpose, the FMEA process closely examines the human-machine interface that is necessary to the successful operation of equipment.

For example, by using this process, health-care providers can predict how and when errors and other failures with infusion pumps may occur. It works by gathering an interdisciplinary team (e.g., nurses, physicians, pharmacists, engineering staff, risk and quality staff) to identify as many errors and other failures that could possibly occur when using the pump, and to predict how harmful these failures could be. The goal is to prevent poor results so, of course, the process includes taking action to eliminate, or at least reduce, the risk of failures that could harm patients.

The following questions can be used to begin discussions about the potential sources of failure with infusion pumps.

Using FMEA to Predict Failures with Infusion Pumps[26]

I. Basic Functionality—How well does the pump perform the required task?

a. Is this the correct pump to perform the desired task(s)?

b. Can the pump deliver the volume/increments needed under the correct pressure?

c. Are any features incompatible with the environment where it will be used (e.g., size, weight, number of channels)?

d. Will the pump deliver medications in the concentrations most typically used?

e. What tubing and other supplies are required for the pump to perform effectively and safely? Are they interchangeable with other pumps? Could interchangeable tubing be used for this pump, rendering it unsafe?

f. Are users alerted to pump-setting errors? Wrong patient errors? Wrong channel errors? Wrong medication/solution errors? Mechanical failure?

g. Does the pump have memory functions for settings and alarms with an easily retrievable log? If the pump is turned off, does it retain settings for a period of time?

II. User-Machine Interface—How easy and intuitive is it for people to use the pump?

a. What functionalities do users expect the pump to have?

b. Is the number of steps for programming minimal?

c. Are the touch buttons used for programming clearly labeled, logically positioned, and the proper size?

d. Are the screens readable with proper font size, lighting, contrast, and other cues to enhance performance?

e. Do the units of medication delivery (e.g., mcg/kg, mcg/kg/min) match current practices?

f. Do the medications, units of delivery, and strengths appear in a logical sequence for selection?

g. Is there any information that defaults to a predetermined value? If yes, is it safe?

h. Is it easy to install and prime administration sets, and to remove air in the line?

i. Are any special features such as drug/dose calculations and dose alerts helpful and easy to use?

j. Are the screens free of abbreviations, trailing zeros (e.g., 1.0 mg), and naked decimal points (e.g., .1mg)?

k. Do the alarms clearly guide staff to the problems? Is it possible to permanently disable audible alarms, or set them too low to be heard?

l. If the infusion rate is changed, but not confirmed, does the device continuously alert the user that the solution is infusing at the old rate?

m. Could the administration sets be mispositioned during installation, or accidentally dislodged, separated, or removed by patients?

n. Does the administration set prevent gravity free-flow of the solution when it is removed from the pump?

o. Is the device tamper resistant?

p. Does the pump fit into the typical workflow?

q. How does the pump compare to the pumps now in use?

Error
Reporting

DEFINE MEDICATION ERRORS[36]

A medication error is any preventable event that may cause or lead to inappropriate medication use or to patient harm while the medication is in the control of the healthcare professional, patient, or consumer. Such events may be related to professional practice, healthcare products, procedures, and systems, including prescribing; order communication; product labeling, packaging, and nomenclature; compounding; dispensing; distribution; administration; education; monitoring; and use.

WHY REPORT ERRORS?

Event reporting is the primary means through which an organization **learns** about:

- Potential risks—risks hidden in the processes used to provide patient care
- Actual errors—errors that occur during patient care
- Causes of errors—underlying weaknesses in the systems and processes of care that explain why an error happened
- Prevention—ways to prevent recurrent events and, ultimately, patient harm

The only way to achieve medication safety is to **look** for risks that could lead to a medication error, and to **learn** from errors that actually occur. Nurses are often in the best position to detect an actual medication error, especially if it originates during the prescribing or dispensing of medications. The next step is to report hazardous conditions and errors and **learn** from the reports of others to prevent future errors.

WHERE TO REPORT ERRORS?

Internal Reporting

The facility in which you work will ask you to report all errors to your nurse/risk manager. Your facility should have an error reporting policy that specifies the types of events to report. No matter how insignificant an incident may seem, immediate reporting is always the best approach. If an error reached the patient (including omitted medications), check with your manager about documenting the event in the patient's medical record. A good rule of thumb is to document the factual event without going into detail about the underlying causes. However, do not document that an event report has been completed.

External Reporting

In addition to reporting errors to your workplace, consider voluntarily reporting errors to outside organizations. You may potentially preventing a harmful error from affecting others. Patient names should not be included in the report. The name of the reporter/facility will remain confidential, but the information learned will be shared with healthcare practitioners, drug manufacturers, equipment and technology vendors, the FDA, and others who can help redesign systems/processes.

Report particularly hazardous conditions or interesting medication errors to:

- Institute for Safe Medication Practices: 1-800-FAIL-SAF(E); www.ismp.org/Pages/communications.asp
- USP-ISMP Medication Errors Reporting Program: www.usp.org/prn
- Food and Drug Administration: 1-800-FDA-1088; www.fda.gov/medwatch

Risk—Hazardous conditions that could lead to an error

- Risks identified during medication administration (e.g., look-alike products, ambiguous product labels, staffing shortages, noise, poor lighting, clutter)

Near Misses—Errors that do not reach the patient

- Errors that are intercepted during prescribing, dispensing, or administering a medication, and are corrected before they reach the patient

Errors, No Harm—Errors that reach the patient but do not cause harm

- No change in patient monitoring is required as a result of the error

Errors, Harm—Errors that reach the patient and cause harm

- Includes any change in the level of care provided as a result of the error

WHAT TO INCLUDE?

The most informative error reports include the following information:

- How an error happened, or the conditions that led to a potential hazard, provided as a narrative description
- Why the error or hazardous condition occurred (the system causes)
- Suggestions for how systems or processes can be changed to prevent similar errors involving other staff

The following is a sample medication error-reporting format, which quickly gathers the causative factors through use of basic probing questions.

Medication System Analyze-ERR™

Incident #: _____

Patient MR# (if error reached patient)		
Date of error: _____	Date information obtained: _____	Patient age: _____

Drug(s) involved in error: _____

Non-formulary drug(s)?	Yes	No
Drug sample(s)?	Yes	No
Drug(s) packaged in unit dose/unit of use?	Yes	No
Drug(s) dispensed from pharmacy?	Yes	No
Error within 24 hours of admission, transfer, or after discharge?	Yes	No
Did the error reach the patient?	Yes	No

Source of IV solution: □ Manufacturer premixed solution □ Pharmacy IV admixture □ Nursing IV admixture

Brief description of the event (what, when, and why):

Did the patient require any of the following actions after the error that you would not have done if the event had not occurred? □ Testing □ Additional observation □ Gave antidote □ Care escalated (transferred, etc.)
□ Additional LOS □ Other_____

Patient outcome:

Possible causes	Y/N	Comments
Critical patient information missing? (age, weight, allergies, VS, lab values, pregnancy, patient identity, location, renal/liver impairment, diagnoses, etc.)		

Critical drug information missing? (outdated/absent references, inadequate computer screening, inaccessible pharmacist, uncontrolled drug formulary, etc.)

Miscommunication of drug order? (illegible, ambiguous, incomplete, misheard, or misunderstood orders, intimidation/faulty interaction, etc.)

Drug name, label, packaging problem? (look/sound-alike names, look-alike packaging, unclear/absent labeling, faulty drug identification, etc.)

Drug storage or delivery problem? (slow turnaround time, inaccurate delivery, doses missing or expired, multiple concentrations, placed in wrong bin, etc.)

Drug delivery device problem? (poor device design, misprogramming, free-flow, mixed up lines, IV administration of oral syringe contents, etc.)

Environmental, staffing, or workflow problems? (lighting, noise, clutter, interruptions, staffing deficiencies, workload, inefficient workflow, employee safety, etc.)

Lack of staff education? (competency validation, new or unfamiliar drugs/devices, orientation process, feedback about errors/prevention, etc.)

Patient education problem? (lack of information, noncompliance, not encouraged to ask questions, lack of investigating patient inquiries, etc.)

Lack of quality control or independent check systems? (equipment quality control checks, independent checks for high-alert drugs/high-risk patient population drugs, etc.)

© 2002 Institute for Safe Medication Practices.

CATEGORIZING MEDICATION ERRORS[37]

Error reports should be categorized according to the severity of the outcome to the patient. Following is a national, standardized tool designed to index and track medication error reports according to patient outcome. An algorithm is also provided to select the proper category for each error report.

For the purpose of learning and change, however, an event report that falls into category **A (no error)** is equally important as an event report in category **I (error, harm)**. Therefore, *all* reports should be fully investigated and acted upon to reduce the risk of errors.

NCC MERP Index

Definitions

Harm: Impairment of the physical, emotional, or psychological function or structure of the body and/or pain resulting therefrom.

Monitoring: To observe or record relevant physiological or psychological signs.

Intervention: May include change in therapy or active medical/surgical treatment.

Intervention necessary to sustain life: Includes cardiovascular and respiratory support (e.g., CPR, defibrillation, intubation).

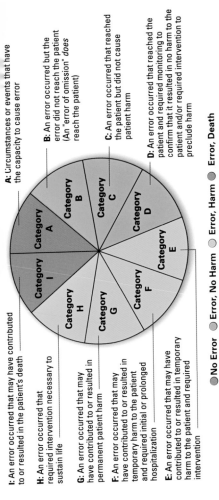

A: Circumstances or events that have the capacity to cause error

B: An error occurred but the error did not reach the patient (An "error of omission" *does* reach the patient)

C: An error occurred that reached the patient but did not cause patient harm

D: An error occurred that reached the patient and required monitoring to confirm that it resulted in no harm to the patient and/or required intervention to preclude harm

E: An error occurred that may have contributed to or resulted in temporary harm to the patient and required intervention

F: An error occurred that may have contributed to or resulted in temporary harm to the patient and required initial or prolonged hospitalization

G: An error occurred that may have contributed to or resulted in permanent patient harm

H: An error occurred that required intervention necessary to sustain life

I: An error occurred that may have contributed to or resulted in the patient's death

● No Error ● Error, No Harm ○ Error, Harm ● Error, Death

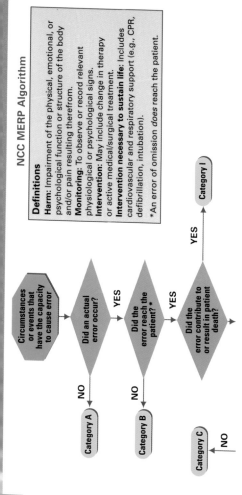

NCC MERP Algorithm

Definitions

Harm: Impairment of the physical, emotional, or psychological function or structure of the body and/or pain resulting therefrom.

Monitoring: To observe or record relevant physiological or psychological signs.

Intervention: May include change in therapy or active medical/surgical treatment.

Intervention necessary to sustain life: Includes cardiovascular and respiratory support (e.g., CPR, defibrillation, intubation).

*An error of omission *does* reach the patient.

Circumstances or events that have the capacity to cause error

Did an actual error occur?

NO → Category A

YES

Did the error reach the patient? *

NO → Category B

YES

Did the error contribute to or result in patient death?

YES → Category I

NO → Category C

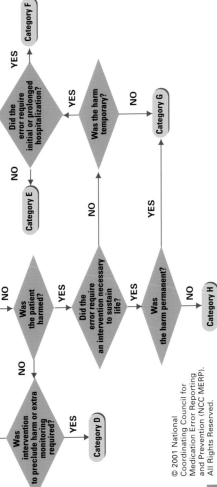

Was the patient harmed?

NO → Was intervention to preclude harm or extra monitoring required?

YES → Category D

YES → Did the error require an intervention necessary to sustain life?

YES → Was the harm permanent?

NO → Category H

YES → Category G

NO → Was the harm temporary?

YES → Did the error require initial or prolonged hospitalization?

NO → Category E

YES → Category F

NO → Category G

113

Key terms highlighted in **green** throughout
the text are defined in the **Glossary**.

ACCESS TO INFORMATION

Improving access to information is one of the key safety principles for safeguarding **high-alert medications**. On a daily basis, nurses need information on a variety of drug-related topics to safely administer medications. For example, while providing morning medications to several patients, a nurse could easily need to reference all of the following:

- Compatibility of a medication with IV solution
- Typical mg/kg dose of a common pediatric analgesic
- Cross allergy between aspirin and another medication
- Appropriate conversion of an IV opioid dose to an oral dose
- Safe rate for an IV push medication
- Safety of crushing a medication
- Rate of infusion for continuous IV heparin

A reliable up-to-date drug reference text or electronic database is a must. However, up-to-date quick reference tables provide an additional way to ensure that nurses have ready access to commonly needed information. Dose-related reference charts can also eliminate the need for error-prone mathematical calculations.

A variety of selected reference tables are provided, which can be used to maximize patient safety during drug administration.

Syringe Compatibility Chart[35]

	Atropine	Buprenorphine	Butorphanol	Chlorpromazine	Cimetidine	Codeine	Diazepam	Dimenhydrinate	Diphenhydramine	Droperidol	Fentanyl	Glycopyrrolate	Haloperidol Lactate
Thiethylperazine				C									
Secobarbital					—								
Scopolamine HBr	C		C	C	C			C	C	C	C	C	C
Ranitidine	C		C	—	—		—	C	C	C	C	C	C
Promethazine	C		C	C	C			—	C	C	C	C	C
Procaine	C		C	C	C			—	C	C	C	C	C
Prochlorperazine	C		C	C	C			—	C	C	C	C	C
Perphenazine	C		C	C	C				C	C	C	C	C
Pentobarbital	C		—	C	C			C	—	—	—	—	—
Pentazocine	C		C	C	C			C	C	C	C	—	
Nalbuphine	C			C				—	C	C	C	C	
Morphine	C		C	C	C			C	C	C	C	C	
Midazolam	C	C	C	C	C			—	C	C	C	C	
Metoclopramide	C		C	C	C			C	C	C	C	C	
Meperidine	C		C	C	C			C	C	C	C	C	
Hydroxyzine	C		C	C	C	C		—	C	C	C	C	—
Heparin	C			—	C			—	C		—	C	—
Haloperidol Lactate								—	—		—	—	
Glycopyrrolate	C		C	C	C	C		—	C	C			
Fentanyl	C		C	C	C			C	C	C			
Droperidol	C		C	C	C			C	C	C	C		
Diphenhydramine	C		C	C	C			C	—				
Dimenhydrinate	C		—	—				C	C	C	—	—	
Diazepam	C		C										
Codeine	C												
Cimetidine	C												
Chlorpromazine	C	C		—									
Butorphanol	C												
Buprenorphine													
Atropine													

Syringe Compatibility Table (continued)

	Heparin	Hydroxyzine	Meperidine	Metoclopramide	Midazolam	Morphine	Nalbuphine	Pentazocine	Pentobarbital	Perphenazine	Prochlorperazine	Promazine	Promethazine	Ranitidine	Scopolamine HBr
Heparin															
Hydroxyzine	C														
Meperidine	C	C													
Metoclopramide	C	C	C												
Midazolam	C	C	C	C											
Morphine	C	C	C	C	C										
Nalbuphine	C	C	C	I	C	C									
Pentazocine	C	I	C	C	C	C	I								
Pentobarbital	C	I	I	I	I	I	I	I							
Perphenazine	C	C	C	C	C	C	C	C	I						
Prochlorperazine	C	C	C	C	C	C	C	C	I	C					
Promazine	C	C	C	C	C	C	C	C	I	C	C				
Promethazine	C	C	C	C	C	C	C	C	I	C	C	C			
Ranitidine	C	C	C	C	C	C	C	I	C	C	C	C	C		
Scopolamine HBr	C	C	C	C	C	C	C	C	I	C	C	C	C	C	
Secobarbital		I							I					I	I
Thiethylperazine	C	C			C					C	C		C	C	C

C, compatible; I, incompatible; □, no documented information.

The syringe compatibility table provides physical compatibility information only for drugs mixed in a syringe. Therapeutic incompatibilities are not represented, therefore, professional judgement should be exercised when utilizing this table.

SOLUTION COMPATIBILITY CHART[6]

Intravenous Medication	D5W	D10W	D5/¼NS	D5/½NS	D5NS	NS	½NS	R	LR	D5LR
Acetazolamide	C	C	C	C	C	C	C	C	C	C
Acyclovir	C		C	C	C	C			C	
Aminophylline	C	C	C	C	C	C	C	C	C	C
Antithymocyte Globulin	C	C	C	C	C	C	C			
Ascorbic Acid	C	C	C	C	C	C	C	C	C	C
Aztreonam	C	C	C	C	C	C		C	C	C
Calcium Chloride	C	C	C	C	C	C		C	C	C
Calcium Gluconate	C	C			C	C			C	C
Cefazolin	C	C	C	C	C	C		C	C	C
Cefoperazone	C	C			C	C			C	
Cefotaxime	C	C	C	C	C	C			C	
Cefotetan	C					C				
Cefoxitin	C	C	C	C	C	C		C	C	C
Ceftazidime	C	C	C	C	C	C		C	C	C
Ceftizoxime	C	C	C	C	C	C		C	C	
Ceftriaxone	C	C		C		C				
Cefuroxime	C	C	C	C	C	C		C	C	
Cimetidine	C	C	C	C	C	C		C	C	C
Clindamycin	C	C		C	C	C			C	
Dexamethasone	C					C				
Dobutamine	C	C		C	C	C	C		C	C
Dopamine	C	C		C	C	C			C	C
Doxycycline	C				C	C		C		
Epinephrine	C	C	C	C	C	C		C	C	C
Famotidine	C	C				C			C	
Fentanyl	C					C				

Intravenous Medication	D5W	D10W	D5/1/4NS	D5/1/2NS	D5NS	NS	1/2NS	R	LR	D5LR
Folic Acid	C					C				
Furosemide	C	C			C	C			C	C
Gentamicin	C	C				C		C	C	
Heparin NA			C	C	C	C	C	C		C
Hydrocortisone Phosphate	C	C				C		C		
Hydrocortisone Na Succinate	C	C	C	C	C	C	C	C	C	C
Hydromorphone	C	C			C	C	C	C	C	C
Imipenem-Cilastatin	C[4]	C[4]	C[4]	C[4]	C[4]	C[10]				
Insulin (Regular)	C[P]	C		C		C[P]			C	
Isoproterenol	C[P]	C	C	C	C	C[P]		C	C	C
Kanamycin	C	C			C	C			C	
Labetalol	C		C		C	C	C		C	C
Lidocaine	C[P]			C	C	C	C		C	C
Magnesium Sulfate	C					C			C	
Meperidine	C	C	C	C	C	C	C	C	C	C
Meropenem	C[1]	C[1]	C[1]		C[1]	C[4]		C[4]	C[4]	C[1]
Metoclopramide	C			C		C			C	C
Morphine	C	C			C	C			C	C
Multivitamin	C	C				C			C	C
Nafcillin Na	C	C	C	C	C	C		C	C	C
Nitroglycerin	C				C	C	C			C	C
Norepinephrine	C[P]				C[P]	C				
Ondansetron	C				C	C	C			
Oxacillin	C	C			C				C	C
Pancuronium	C				C	C			C	
Papaverine	C	C	C	C	C	C	C	C		
Penicillin G, K	C	C	C	C	C	C	C	C	C	C

Continued

Solution Compatibility (continued)

Intravenous Medication	D5W	D10W	D5/¼NS	D5/½NS	D5NS	NS	½NS	R	LR	D5LR
Pentobarbital	C	C	C	C	C	C	C	C	C	C
Piperacillin/ Tazobactam	C				C	C				
Potassium Acetate	C	C				C			C	C
Potassium Chloride	C	C	C	C	C	C	C	C	C	C
Potassium Phosphate	C	C	C	C	C	C	C			
Prochlorperazine	C	C	C	C	C	C	C	C	C	C
Propranolol	C[P]			C	C	C	C		C	
Pyridoxine	C	C	C	C	C	C		C	C	
Ranitidine	C	C		C		C			C	
Sodium Acetate	C	C			C	C	C	C		C
Sodium Bicarbonate	C	C	C	C	C	C	C			
Sodium Chloride	C	C	C	C	C	C	C	C	C	C
Succinylcholine	C	C	C	C	C	C	C	C	C	C
Thiamine	C	C	C	C	C	C	C	C	C	C
Thiopental	C		C	C	C[6]	C	C			
Trace Metals	C	C			C	C			C	
Tranexamic Acid	C	C	C	C	C	C		C		
Warfarin	C	C		C	C	C				C
Zidovudine	C[P]					C				

KEY

C	= Compatible*	R	= Ringer's solution
W	= Compatible in water not NS	D5LR	= 5% Dextrose in Lactated Ringer's solution
D5W	= 5% Dextrose in water	1	= Stable for 1 hour
D10W	= 10% Dextrose in water	2	= Stable for 2 hours
D5/¼ NS	= 5% Dextrose in ¼ normal saline	4	= Stable for 4 hours
D5/½ NS	= 5% Dextrose in ½ normal saline	6	= Stable for 6 hours
D5NS	= 5% Dextrose in normal saline	10	= Stable for 10 hours
½ NS	= ½ Normal saline	P	= Preferred diluent

*Compatibility in various concentrations may vary; consult pharmacist.

IM Use Only Medications[11]

The following medications can only be administered intramuscularly (IM).

GENERIC	BRAND
betamethasone sodium phosphate & acetate	Celestone Soluspan
corticotropin zinc hydroxide	Cortrophin Zinc
dexamethasone acetate	Dalalone L.A., etc.
dicyclomine HCl injection	Bentyl
dimercaprol	BAL in Oil
estradiol cypionate (in oil)	Depo-estradiol, etc.
estradiol valerate (in oil)	Delestrogen, etc.
estrone	Kestrone
fluphenazine decanoate	Prolixin
haloperidol decanoate	Haldol
hydrocortisone acetate	Hydrocortone
hydroxocobalamine, crystalline	Vitamin B$_{12}$
hydroxyprogesterone caproate (in oil)	Hylutin
hydroxyzine injection	Vistaril
leuprolide acetate depot	Lupron
medroxyprogesterone acetate	Depo-Provera
methylprednisolone acetate injection	Depo-Medrol, etc.
nandrolone decanoate	Deca-Durabolin, etc.
nandrolone phenpropionate	Durabolin, etc.
penicillin G procaine	Wycillin
penicillin G benzathine	Bicillin L-A, etc.
prednisolone acetate injection	Key-Pred 25 etc.
progesterone injection (in oil)	Progesterone
rabies vaccine	Imovax
testosterone injection	many
triamcinolone diacetate	Aristocort, etc.
triamcinolone hexacetonide	Aristospan

As a general rule, vaccines and hormonal agents are typically administered IM and can cause harm if given IV.

Select *Do Not Crush* Medications[31]

General formulations of medications that should not be crushed include:

- Enteric coated medications—drug released too early, may be destroyed by stomach acids or cause irritation
- Extended release formulations—can potentially deliver a toxic dose (abbreviations such as CR, LA, SA, SR, TD, TR, XL, XR)
- Sublingual formulations—designed only to be absorbed rapidly in the mouth
- Carcinogenic/teratogenic medications—can expose handlers to aerosolized medication
- Other—can irritate the oral mucosa, are extremely bitter, can permanently dye or stain teeth and mucosa

Many medications (including some on this list) are available in a liquid suspension formulation. Check with your pharmacist for availability in your institution.

Do Not Crush Medications		
GENERIC NAME	**SELECTED BRAND NAMES**	**RATIONALE**
alendronate	Fosamax	mucosal irritant
amoxicillin/ clavulanate	Augmentin XR	slow release
atomoxetine	Strattera	mucosal irritant
bisacodyl	Dulcolax	enteric coated
buproprion	Wellbutrin SR	slow release
cefuroxime	Ceftin	bitter taste
ciprofloxacin	Cipro	bitter taste
diltiazem	Dilacor XR, Cardizem CD, Cardizem LA, Cardizem SR, Tiazac	slow release

GENERIC NAME	SELECTED BRAND NAMES	RATIONALE
divalproex sodium	Depakote	slow release
divalproex sodium extended release	Depakote ER	slow release
docusate	Colace	bitter taste
ferrous sulfate	Feratab	enteric coated
finasteride	Proscar, Propecia	teratogenic potential
glipizide	Glucotrol XL	slow release
ibuprofen	Motrin	bitter taste
isotretinoin	Accutane	mucosal irritant
lansoprazole	Prevacid	slow release
lithium	Lithobid	slow release
mesalamine	Asacol, Pentasa	slow release
morphine	MS Contin	slow release
mycophenolate mofetil	CellCept	teratogenic potential
nifedipine	Procardia XL	slow release
nitroglycerin	Nitrong, Nitrostat	sublingual formulation
oxybutynin extended-release	Ditropan XL	slow release
propranolol long-acting	Inderal LA, Inderide LA	slow release
valproic acid	Depakene	mucosal irritant, slow release
verapamil	Calan SR, Covera HS, verapamil hydrochloride SR	slow release

Acetaminophen Combination Products

Patients receiving more than 4 grams of acetaminophen daily have developed liver toxicity. There are many prescription analgesics that contain acetaminophen as just one of the ingredients. These products are often prescribed by brand names, not alerting nurses to presence of acetaminophen. Various PRN medications prescribed (often on standing orders) could cumulatively result in toxic amounts of acetaminophen. Use this table as a quick reference for common acetaminophen-containing products. If a drug in question is not on the list, refer to a complete drug reference handbook.

Acetaminophen Combination Products[42]

BRAND NAME	ACETAMINOPHEN	OPIOID	OTHER INGREDIENTS
Aceta w/Codeine	300 mg	codeine 30 mg	
Anexsia 5/500	500 mg	hydrocodone 5 mg	
Anexsia 7.5/650	650 mg	hydrocodone 7.5 mg	
Bancap HC	500 mg	hydrocodone 5 mg	
Co-Gesic	500 mg	hydrocodone 5 mg	
Darvocet-N 100	650 mg	propoxyphene-N 100 mg	
Endocet	325 mg	oxycodone 5 mg	
Fioricet	325 mg	none	butalbital 50 mg caffeine 40 mg
Fioricet w/Codeine	325 mg	codeine 30 mg	butalbital 50 mg caffeine 40 mg
Hydrocet	500 mg	hydrocodone 5 mg	
Hydrogesic	500 mg	hydrocodone 5 mg	
Lenoltec w/Codeine No. 1	300 mg	codeine 8 mg	caffeine 15 mg
Lorcet 10/650	650 mg	hydrocodone 10 mg	
Lorcet Plus	650 mg	hydrocodone 7.5 mg	
Lorcet-HD	500 mg	hydrocodone 10 mg	
Lortab 2.5/500	500 mg	hydrocodone 2.5 mg	
Lortab 5/500	500 mg	hydrocodone 5 mg	

continued

Acetaminophen Combination Products (continued)

BRAND NAME	ACETAMINOPHEN	OPIOID	OTHER INGREDIENTS		
Lortab 7.5/500	500 mg	hydrocodone 7.5 mg			
Lortab 10/500	500 mg	hydrocodone 10 mg			
Lortab Elixir Per 5 mL	167 mg	hydrocodone 2.5 mg			
Medigesic	325 mg	none	butalbital 50 mg	caffeine 40 mg	
Norco	325 mg	hydrocodone 10 mg			
Norco 5/325	325 mg	hydrocodone 5 mg			
Panacet 5/500	500 mg	hydrocodone 5 mg			
Percocet 2.5/325	325 mg	oxycodone 2.5 mg			
Percocet 5/325	325 mg	oxycodone 5 mg			
Percocet 7.5/500	500 mg	oxycodone 7.5 mg			
Percocet 10/650	650 mg	oxycodone 10 mg			
Repan	325 mg	none	butalbital 50 mg	caffeine 40 mg	
Roxicet 5/500	500 mg	oxycodone 5 mg			
Roxicet Oral Solution Per 5 mL	325 mg	oxycodone 5 mg			
Sedapap-10	650 mg	none	butalbital 50 mg		
Talacen	650 mg	pentazocine 25 mg			
T-Gesic	500 mg	hydrocodone 5 mg			

-semide	Diuretics	furosemide (Lasix)	Hypotension; hyperglycemia; electrolyte imbalances; gout
-thiazide	Diuretics	chlorothiazide hydrochlorothiazide	Hypotension; photosensitivity; hypokalemia
-tiazem	Calcium channel blockers	diltiazem (Cardizem)	Gingival hyperplasia; sinus bradycardia; dizziness
-toin	Antiepileptic	phenytoin (Dilantin)	Bradycardia; gingival hyperplasia; hypertrichosis
-triptan	Antimigraine agents	sumatriptan (Imitrex)	Chest pain/tightness; flushing; myalgia
-triptyline	Antidepressants	amitriptyline	Sedation; hypotension; restlessness
-vastatin	Antihyperlipidemic	atorvastatin (Lipitor)	Arthralgia; weakness; mild myalgia

Dopamine Infusion Rate Chart[34]
400 mg in 250 mL or 800 mg in 500 mL
(1600 mcg/mL concentration)

Find your patient's body weight in the first row. Then locate the ordered infusion rate in mcg/kg/min in the left column. The intersecting cell will be the mL/h infusion rate.

Ordered Infusion Rate (mcg/kg/min)	Patient Body Weight (kg)									
	10	20	30	40	50	60	70	80	90	100
2.5	1	2	3	4	5	6	7	8	8	9
5	2	4	6	8	9	11	13	15	17	19
10	4	8	11	15	19	22	26	30	34	38
15	6	11	17	23	28	34	40	45	51	56
20	8	15	23	30	38	45	53	60	68	75
25	9	19	28	38	47	56	66	75	84	94
30	11	23	34	45	56	68	79	90	101	113
35	13	26	39	53	65	79	92	105	118	131
40	15	30	45	60	75	90	105	120	135	150
45	17	34	51	68	84	101	118	135	152	169
50	19	38	56	75	94	113	131	150	169	188

BASICS

SEE ALSO

> HIGH-ALERT DRUGS

Basics

DOSE CALCULATORS

Dosages

$$\frac{\text{Dose ordered}}{\text{Dose on hand}} = \text{Amount to administer}$$

Example: Tablet $\dfrac{15 \text{ mg}}{5 \text{ mg/tablet}} = 3 \text{ tablets}$

Liquid $\dfrac{35 \text{ mg}}{50 \text{ mg/mL}} = 0.7 \text{ mL}$

Solution Concentration

$$\frac{\text{Dosage in solution}}{\text{Volume of solution}} = \text{Solution concentration}$$

Example: $\dfrac{100 \text{ mg}}{500 \text{ mL}} = 0.2 \text{ mg/mL}$

IV Dose Rate Calculation

$$\frac{\text{Dose ordered}}{\text{Solution concentration}} = \text{Volume/hour}$$

Example: $\dfrac{50 \text{ mg/hr}}{2 \text{ mg/mL}} = 25 \text{ mL/hr}$

HEIGHT AND WEIGHT CONVERSION

Height	1 in = 2.54 cm; 1 cm = 0.3937 in		
in	cm	cm	in
1	2.5	1	0.4
2	5.1	2	0.8
4	10.2	3	1.2
6	15.2	4	1.6
8	20.3	5	2.0
10	25.4	6	2.4
20	50.8	8	3.1
30	76.2	10	3.9
40	101.6	20	7.9
50	127.0	30	11.8
60	152.4	40	15.7
70	177.8	50	19.7
80	203.2	60	23.6
90	227.6	70	27.6
100	254.0	80	31.5
150	381.0	90	35.4
200	508.0	100	39.4

Weight	1 lb = 0.454 kg; 1 kg = 2.204 lb		
lb	kg	kg	lb
1	0.5	1	2.2
2	0.9	2	4.4
4	1.8	3	6.6
6	2.7	4	8.8
8	3.6	5	11.0
10	4.5	6	13.2
20	9.1	8	17.6
30	13.6	10	22
40	18.1	20	44
50	22.7	30	66
60	27.2	40	88
70	31.8	50	110
80	36.3	60	132
90	40.9	70	154
100	45.4	80	176
150	68.0	90	198
200	90.7	100	220

Insulin Administration

Tips[30A]

- Route is subcutaneous.*
- Angle of administration is 45-90 degrees.
- Injection goes in the subcutaneous tissue.
- Insulin sites should be rotated.

Recommendations for Mixing Insulins[39]

- When mixing short- and long-acting insulins in the same syringe, draw up the short-acting insulin first and then the long-acting insulin.
- Patients whose blood sugar levels are well controlled on a mixed-insulin dose should maintain their individual routine.
- Insulin should not be mixed with other medications.
- Insulin should not be diluted unless approved by the prescriber.
- Rapid-acting insulins that are mixed with neutral protamine Hagedorn (NPH) or Ultralente insulins should be injected 15 minutes before a meal.
- Short-acting and Lente insulins should not be mixed unless the patient's blood sugar level is currently under control with this mixture.

*Regular insulin can be given intravenously.

Common Hypoglycemic Agents[39]

TYPES	PEAK (hr)	DURATION (hr)
Oral agents		
Chlorpropamide (Diabinese)	1	24-60
Tolbutamide (Orinase)	5-8	6-12
Tolazamide (Tolinase)	4-6	12-24
Glipizide (Glucotrol)	1-3	10-24
Glyburide (DiaBeta, Micronase, Glynase PresTab)	2-8	24
Acarbose (Precose)	1	14-24
Acetohexamide (Dymelor)	1.3-8	12-24
Glimepiride (Amaryl)	2-3	24
Metformin hydrochloride (Glucophage)	1-3	9-17
Miglitol (Glyset)	2-3	24
Nateglinide (Starlix)	0-1	2-3
Repaglinide (Prandin)	1-1.5	<4
Insulin		
Rapid acting (onset 15 min-1 hr)		
Regular	2-4	4-12
Insulin zinc (Semilente)	5-10	12-16
Regular human (Humulin-R, Novolin-R)	1-3	3-5
Intermediate acting (onset 2-4 hr)		
Globin zinc (Iletin)	6-10	18-24
Isophane suspension (NPH)	4-12	18-24
Insulin zinc suspension (Iletin Lente)	7-15	18-24
NPH human isophane (Humulin-N, Novolin-N)	8-12	26-30
Long acting (onset 4-6 hr)		
Protamine zinc (PZ)	14-24	24-36
Insulin zinc extended (Ultralente)	10-30	>36
Insulin glargine (Lantus)	N/A	24

N/A, not applicable; **NPH**, neutral protamine Hagedorn.

Adult Sites, Needle Sizes, and Volume for IM, Subcut, ID Injections[4]

TYPE: IM
NEEDLE SIZE
23-25 G
5/8"-1"

VOLUME
Average
0.5 mL
Range
0.5-2 mL

SITE: Deltoid muscle[7]

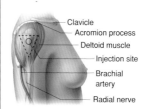

- Clavicle
- Acromion process
- Deltoid muscle
- Injection site
- Brachial artery
- Radial nerve

TYPE: IM
NEEDLE SIZE
20-23 G
1½"-3"

VOLUME

Average
2 mL
Range
1-5 mL

SITE: Ventrogluteal muscle[7]

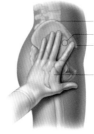

- Iliac crest
- Injection site
- Anterior superior iliac spine
- Greater trochanter of femur

TYPE: IM
NEEDLE SIZE
20-23 G
1½"-3"

VOLUME
Average
2 mL
Range
1-5 mL

SITE: Dorsogluteal muscle[7]

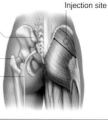

- Injection site
- Posterior superior iliac spine
- Greater trochanter of femur
- Sciatic nerve

	SITE: Vastus lateralis muscle[7]
TYPE: IM **NEEDLE SIZE** 22-25 G 5/8″–1 1/2″ **VOLUME** **Average** 2 mL **Range** 1-5 mL	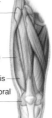 Greater trochanter of femur Injection site (middle third) Vastus lateralis Lateral femoral condyle
TYPE: Subcut **NEEDLE SIZE** 25-27 G 1/2″–5/8″ **VOLUME** **Average** 0.5 mL **Range** 0.5-1.5 mL	**SITE:** Arm, abdomen, thigh[7] 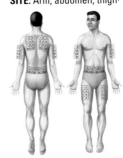
TYPE: ID **NEEDLE SIZE** 26-27 G 3/8″ **VOLUME** **Average** 0.1 mL **Range** 0.001-1.0 mL	**SITE:** Forearm[7] 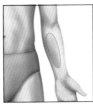

Pediatric IM Injection Sites[3A]

Age	Preferred Muscle Group	Needle Length
Infant less than 4 mo	Ventrogluteal or vastus lateralis	$5/8$-$7/8$ in
Infant 4 mo and older	Ventrogluteal or vastus lateralis	$5/8$-1 in
Toddler	Ventrogluteal or dorsogluteal over 3 yr and walking for 1 yr	$5/8$-1 in
Older child	Deltoid or ventrogluteal	$5/8$-1 in

Vastus Lateralis Intramuscular Injection Site—Lateral Thigh[7]

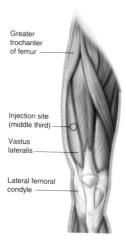

Greater trochanter of femur

Injection site (middle third)

Vastus lateralis

Lateral femoral condyle

Z-Track Injection[7]

Purpose: Prevents seepage of medication through injection track with an IM injection.

1. Prepare injection.
2. Select site.
3. Clean skin with alcohol.
4. Slide skin to side 1–1.5 in.
5. Inject medication at 90-degree angle.
6. Withdraw needle.
7. Release skin.

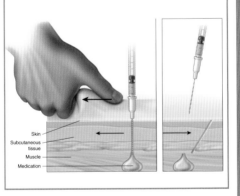

Skin
Subcutaneous tissue
Muscle
Medication

Preferred Sites for Intravenous Access in Infants[32]

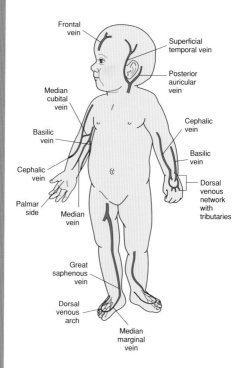

Frontal vein

Superficial temporal vein

Posterior auricular vein

Median cubital vein

Cephalic vein

Basilic vein

Basilic vein

Cephalic vein

Dorsal venous network with tributaries

Palmar side

Median vein

Great saphenous vein

Dorsal venous arch

Median marginal vein

Recommended Childhood and Adolescent Immunization Schedule — United States, 2004

	range of recommended ages				catch-up vaccination				preadolescent assessment		
Vaccine ▼ Age ▶	Birth	1 mo	2 mos	4 mos	6 mos	12 mos	15 mos	18 mos	24 mos	4-6 yrs	11-12 yrs	13-18 yrs
Hepatitis B	HepB #1 only if mother HBsAg (−)	HepB #2	HepB #2		HepB #3						HepB series	
Diphtheria, Tetanus, Pertussis			DTaP	DTaP	DTaP		DTaP	DTaP		DTaP	Td	Td
Haemophilus influenzae Type b			Hib	Hib	Hib	Hib	Hib					
Inactivated Polio			IPV	IPV	IPV		IPV			IPV		
Measles, Mumps, Rubella						MMR #1	MMR #1			MMR #2	MMR #2	
Varicella						Varicella	Varicella		Varicella		Varicella	
Pneumococcal			PCV	PCV	PCV	PCV	PCV		PCV	PPV		
Hepatitis A									Hepatitis A series			
Influenza					Influenza (yearly)							

Vaccines below this line are for selected populations

■ Indicates catch-up vaccine

Any dose not given at recommended time should be given at any subsequent visit. Consult www.cdc.gov and the manufacturer's package for full details.

145

Recommended Adult Immunization Schedule, United States, 2003-2004

Legend	
For all persons in this group	Catch-up on childhood vaccinations
For persons with medical indications	

Vaccine	19-49 Years	50-64 Years	65 Years and Older
Tetanus, Diphtheria (Td)	1 dose booster every 10 years		
Influenza	1 annual dose	1 annual dose	
Pneumococcal	1 dose		1 dose
Hepatitis B	3 doses (0, 1-2, 4-6 months)		
Hepatitis A	2 doses (0, 6-12 months)		
Measles, Mumps, Rubella (MMR)	1 dose if unreliable vaccine Hx; 2 doses if medically indicated		
Varicella	2 doses (0, 4-8 weeks) for persons who are susceptible		
Meningococcal	1 dose		

For more information, go to www.cdc.gov

146

Accident: An event involving damage to a defined system that disrupts the ongoing or future output of that system.

Adverse drug event: An injury to a patient, which is caused by the use of medications or by the failure to use appropriate medications when indicated, rather than by the patient's underlying condition.

Bar code: A graphic representation of data (alpha, numeric, or both) that is machine readable. It uses narrow bars and spaces to create a code for numbers or alphabetic characters. Scanning a bar code gives instant access to information in an associated database.

Computerized practitioner order entry (CPOE): A networked computerized system that allows healthcare professionals to enter orders online.

Error: An act (intended or unintended) that does not achieve its intended outcome.

Failure: A condition in which a part of a system or a system itself does not behave in the intended way it was designed.

Failure mode: The ways in which errors can potentially occur in a system.

Failure mode and effects analysis (FMEA): An analysis of failure modes (the ways errors occur), their consequences, and their risks, performed before problems occur.

Application of FMEA involves following a medication or drug delivery device from the point of manufacture to its administration to a patient and anticipating all modes of failure that could possibly occur.

Forcing functions: Techniques that reduce the possibility that a medication can be administered in a potentially harmful manner (e.g., giving oral liquid doses in oral syringes that will not fit with IV tubing and to which needles cannot be attached; and computer order entry that can be used to "force" the physician to order standardized products). Often referred to as a lock and key design.

Formulary: Lists of drugs or collections of recipes, formulas, and prescriptions for the compounding of medicinal preparations. Formularies differ from pharmacopoeias in that they are less complete, lacking full descriptions of the drugs, their formulations, analytic composition, chemical properties, etc. In hospitals, formularies list all drugs commonly stocked in the hospital pharmacy.

High-alert medication: Medications that have a higher risk of causing patient injury or death when misused. Although errors may not be more common with these drugs than with others, their consequences of errors may be more devastating.

High-risk patient: Those patients at greater risk for harm in the event of a medication error. Includes, but is not limited to, pediatric and geriatric patients, pregnant and lactating women, and immunocompromised and oncology patients.

Root cause analysis (RCA): A process for identifying the basic or causal factor(s) that underlie the occurrence or possible occurrence of an adverse event. This process happens after an event occurs.

Redundancy: An act of repetition intended to duplicate critical actions and mechanisms; if a system has redundancy, a single failure does not result in loss or error in that action. If two people do the same task independently, the probability that both of them will make the same mistake is small.

System: Interdependent elements (human and non-human) interacting to achieve a common aim.

Systems thinking: An approach to risk prevention that looks at how individual processes connect or are interrelated, and how flaws in the process or "system" may be at the root of many seemingly unrelated events that result or have the potential to result in patient harm.

Tall man lettering: Enhancement of unique letter characters of drug names by use of upper case characters. May also include italics, color background, or a combination of these elements to improve differentiation of look-alike drug names.

Independent double check: A procedure in which two individuals, preferably two licensed practitioners, separately check each component of the work process. An example is one person calculating a medication dose for a specific patient, a second individual independently performing the same calculation (not just verifying the calculation), and then comparing the two results before medication administration.

Medication error: Any preventable event that may cause or lead to inappropriate medication use or patient harm while the medication is in the control of the healthcare professional, patient, or consumer. May be related to professional practice, healthcare products, procedures, and systems (including prescribing, order communications, product labeling, packaging and nomenclature, compounding, dispensing, distribution, administration, education, monitoring, and use).

Medication safety: Freedom from accidental injury during the course of medication use; the use of activities to avoid, prevent, or correct adverse drug events that may result from the use of medications.

Near miss: Can be defined in two ways: 1) An event or situation that could have resulted in an accident, injury, or illness, but did not, either by chance or through timely intervention. 2) A medication error that is discovered and corrected before it reaches the patient. Also referred to as a "close call" or "near hit."

SOURCES

A indicates the material was adapted from
the source cited.
(Sources #9-24, 46-48 are from *ISMP Medication
Safety Alert!®* from the Institute for Safe
Medication Practices, Huntingdon Valley, PA.
#25-27, 44-45 are also from ISMP.)

1. American Hospital Association, Health Research and Educational Trust, ISMP: *Pathways for medication safety,* Chicago, 2002, American Hospital Association, Health Research and Educational Trust, ISMP.
2. Center for Drug Evaluation and Research: *Name Differentiation Project,* Rockville, MD, 2002, Center for Drug Evaluation and Research.
3. Becton-Dickson Media Center: *A guide for managing the pediatric patient: reducing the pain and anxiety of injections,* 1 Becton Dr, Franklin Lakes, NJ, 1998, Becton-Dickson.
4. Clark JB, Queener SF, Karb VB: *Pharmacologic basis for nursing practice,* ed 6, St Louis, 2003, Mosby.
5. Cohen MR, editor: *Medication errors,* Washington, DC, 1999, American Pharmaceutical Association.
6. Gahart: *Intravenous medications* 2003, ed 19, St Louis, 2003, Mosby.
7. Harkreader H: *Fundamentals of nursing: caring and clinical judgment,* St Louis, 2000, Mosby.
8. Health Research and Educational Trust, ISMP: *Pathways for medication safety,* Chicago, 2002, American Hospital Association.
9. Vol 1-9, 2004.
10. The "five rights," 4(7), 1999.
11. Drugs that should be administered intramuscularly ONLY, 2004
http://www.ismp.org/MSAarticles/im_only.html.
12. Instilling a measure of safety into those "whispering down the lane" verbal orders, 6(2), 2001.
13. ISMP list of error-prone abbreviations, symbols, and dose expressions, 8(24), 2003.
http://www.ismp.org/PDF/ErrorProne.pdf
14. ISMP's list of high-alert medications, 8(25), 2003.

15. JCAHO has it right—pharmacists should review all non-urgent drug orders prior to administration, 5(15), 2000.

16. Medication errors reported in the between 2000-2004, Vol 6-9, 2004.

17. Placing limits on drug inventory minimizes errors with automated dispensing equipment, 3(24), 1998.

18. Safety issues with patient controlled analgesia, part I—how errors occur, 8(14), 2003.

19. Safety issues with patient controlled analgesia, part II—how to prevent errors, 8(15), 2003.

20. Should abbreviations derived from a foreign language be used?, 9(9), 2004.

21. Survey of automated dispensing shows need for practice improvements and safer system design, 4(12), 1999.

22. Tricks but no treats: illusions and medication errors, (22), 2002.

23. The virtues of independent double checks—they really are worth your time, 8(5), 2003.

24. What's in a name? Ways to prevent dispensing errors linked to name confusion, 7(12), 2002.

25. *2004 ISMP medication safety self assessment® for hospitals*, 2004.

26. Using FMEA to predict failures with infusion pumps, *ISMP Nurse Advise-ERR®*, 2(2), 2004.

27. *Medication System Analyze-ERR®*, 2004.

28. JCAHO: *Failure mode and effects analysis in health care: proactive risk reduction,* Oakbrook Terrace, IL, 2002, Joint Commission on Accreditation of Healthcare Organizations.

29. JCAHO: *2004 national patient safety goals,* Oakbrook Terrace, IL, 2004, Joint Commission on Accreditation of Healthcare Organizations.

30. Kee JL, Hayes ER: *Pharmacology: a nursing process approach,* ed 4, Philadelphia, 2003, W.B. Saunders Company.

31. Mitchell JE, Leady MA: *Oral dosage forms that should not be crushed: 2004 revision,* Hospital Pharmacy, July, 2004.

32. Hockenberry MJ: *Wong's nursing care of infants and children,* ed 7, St Louis, 2003, Mosby.

34. Mosby's Drug Consult: *1600 mcg/ml dosing chart for dopamine (ml/h) infusion rate,* St Louis, 2004, Mosby.

35. Mosby's Drug Consult: *Syringe compatibility table,* St Louis, 2004, Mosby. Based on information in Trissel, LA: Handbook on injectable drugs, 11th ed., American Society of Health-System Pharmacists, Inc., Maryland, 2001.

36. National Coordinating Council for Medication Error Reporting and Prevention: *About medication errors,* Rockville, MD, 2004, National Coordinating Council for Medication Error Reporting and Prevention.

37. National Coordinating Council for Medication Error Reporting and Prevention: *NCC MERP Index for categorizing medication errors,* Rockville, MD, 2004, National Coordinating Council for Medication Error Reporting and Prevention.

38. Perry AG et al: *Pocket guide to basic skills and procedures,* ed 5, St Louis, 2003, Mosby.

39. Peterson V: *Just the facts: a pocket guide to basic nursing,* ed 3, St Louis, 2003, Mosby.

42. Skidmore-Roth L: Mosby's 2005 Nursing Drug Reference, St Louis, 2005, Mosby.

43. USAN Council: *Newly approved USAN stems,* Chicago, 2004, American Medical Association.

44. All is not as it seems…Based on this order, how often should Lovenox be given?, *ISMP Nurse Advise-ERR®,* 2(7), 2004.

45. All is not as it seems…Is this heparin order for 25 units per hour?, *ISMP Nurse Advise-ERR®,* 2(1), 2004.

46. Missing the point, 2(22), 1997.

47. Safety briefs, 6(15), 2001.

48. Safety briefs, 7(20), 2002.

INDEX

GLOSSARY

The key terms highlighted in **green** in this **Glossary** are also highlighted throughout the text.